Contents

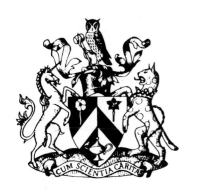

OCCASIONAL PAPER **73**

Needs Assessment in General Practice

S J GILLAM MA, MSc, MRCP, MRCGP, MFPHM
Consultant in Public Health Medicine
Bedfordshire Health Authority

Honorary Senior Lecturer
Department of Epidemiology and Public Health
St Mary's Hospital Medical School, University of London

S A MURRAY MD, MRCGP
General Practitioner
Edinburgh

Senior Lecturer
Department of General Practice
University of Edinburgh

Published by
The Royal College of General Practitioners

October 1996

The Royal College of General Practitioners

Charter

The Royal College of General Practitioners was founded in 1952, with this object:

"To encourage, foster, and maintain the highest possible standards in general medical practice and for that purpose to take or join with others in taking steps consistent with the charitable nature of that object which may assist towards the same."

Among its responsibilities under its Royal Charter the College is entitled to:

"Encourage the publication by general medical practitioners of research into medical or scientific subjects with a view to the improvement of general medical practice in any field and to undertake or assist others in undertaking such research.

"Diffuse information on all matters affecting general medical practice and establish, print, publish, issue and circulate such papers, journals, magazines, books, periodicals, and publications and hold such meetings, conferences, seminars, and instructional courses as may assist the object of the College."

College Headquarters

The headquarters of the Royal College is at 14 Princes Gate, Hyde Park, London SW7 1PU (Telephone: 0171-581-3232). Enquiries should be addressed to the General Manager.

Exeter Publications Office

The Publications Office publishes on behalf of the College the series of *Policy Statements*, *Reports from General Practice*, *Occasional Papers*, and books and booklets. It also co-ordinates material for the *RCGP Members' Reference Book*. Enquiries are welcomed and should be addressed to the Honorary Editor, 9 Marlborough Road, Exeter, Devon EX2 4TJ (Telephone: 01392 57938).

Occasional Papers

The *Occasional Paper* series was established in 1976 to offer authors the opportunity to publish manuscripts too long for publication as articles and too short for books. They are assessed for academic acceptability by members of the Editorial Board and other professionals with special interests. Readers should note that they express the views of the authors, and not the College, unless otherwise stated.

The *Occasional Papers* are included in *Index Medicus*.

Copyright

First impression 1996
Second impression 1997

Editor's preface

At a time when general practice is facing a substantial problem in morale and the biggest recruitment crisis for thirty years, the acceptance of another major responsibility for which doctors have not been systematically trained does not immediately leap to the forefront of general practitioner priorities. Furthermore this new responsibility, needs assessment in general practice, appears complicated, possibly part of another medical discipline, requiring a numerical approach to thinking, and politically sensitive. Like all new tasks, it is likely to eat up time. Why then should general practitioners consider doing it?

Up to the mid-point of the twentieth century doctors mainly worked alone and responded to requests from individual patients. In many countries, over two-thirds of general practitioners still work alone in the 1990s. Group practice in its present form is most highly developed in the United Kingdom where multidisciplinary teams working from purpose-planned premises are more common than in most other Western countries.

Following the 1911 Lloyd George Act, working men registered with general practitioners and the great majority of their families saw the same family doctor, most commonly through friendly societies and local "clubs". This system was consolidated into a practice population list with the introduction of the National Health Service in 1948 and from then on British general practitioners had the particular advantage of knowing the number of their patients, and their age-sex and geographical distribution. Thanks to the Royal College of General Practitioners a series of instruments was invented which enabled practitioners for the first time to take a population view of their patients rather than seeing them only as individuals. Watts' (1958) description of the age-sex register was followed by Eimerl's (1960) diagnostic index, and the Birmingham Research Unit in particular developed techniques enabling general practitioners to understand and analyse the morbidity and mortality of their registered patients as a group.

It is sometimes said that the population approach to general practice is in some way antagonistic to the personal doctor approach. However, family doctors have always seen patients in the context of family groups, and reviewing groups of patients with a common disease is a long tradition in both generalist and specialist medicine. The advantages have been described by Gray et al. (1994) as "living epidemiology", because the general practice computer database is the most up to date in the National Health Service.

National morbidity surveys show that 95% of the whole population consult a doctor every five years; the typical general practitioner who has been in a practice for 12–15 years will have had personal experience of having met virtually all his/her registered patients and will, through having had seven or eight thousand consultations a year, be able to identify by sheer clinical experience conditions that are common and those that are serious; and living in the community, as most doctors still do, gives general practitioners a shrewd grip of the morbidity patterns within it. This reaches the greatest fulfilment in rural practice where virtually the whole community can be registered with a single practice. The logic of the general practitioner as the professional proxy purchasing for groups of patients came to political fulfilment in the general practitioner contract of 1990, underpinned by the Secretary of State's (1989) paper, *Working for Patients*. If, then, general practitioners do have a good working knowledge of the major problems, is this enough? Is there any need to add a new layer of scientific rigour to the assessment of what patients want or need, and is it really practical in ordinary NHS settings?

Needs assessment

The drive for needs assessment came from three sources. First the profession itself has led the way and sought to maximize the strengths of British general practice with professionally trained generalists, multidisciplinary teams, registered lists and now one of the highest uses of desk top computers in the world. There are remarkable opportunities for assessing the needs of populations registered with practices, and academic general practitioners and public health physicians have led the way.

A second pressure has been from government through the Department of Health. As public funds become increasingly squeezed, the need to focus NHS resources where they are most needed and most effective has become stronger. The call for rationality is increasingly heard.

Thirdly, as society becomes more consumerist, and as the patient's voice becomes louder (reflected perhaps most dramatically by the new composition of the General Medical Council, which in November 1996 will have a quarter of its members lay), so patients themselves want unmet needs addressed and expect the Health Service to be ever more professional. We have to ask ourselves:

- What do patients most need?

- What forms of care are most effective?

Among the techniques available to answer these questions are door-to-door surveys of morbidity, which are particularly good for finding out gaps, particularly amongst patients who are not registered with practitioners. However, interviewers can never find everybody at home and the surveys therefore have a 'decline' rate that is greater than the contact rate with British general practice. A second technique is to use consumer surveys. They can be done by post, by telephone, or face to face, and can ask patients about what they themselves see as their main needs and priorities. Thirdly, there are the conventional mortality statistics published by the Department of Health, now available in detail by health authority, by enumeration districts and even by post codes. But these surveys are better for death rates than for disease.

The changing prevalence of disease such as, for example, the doubling of asthma in the population is still best shown by morbidity surveys in general practice. Despite all the computer techniques and advances in laboratory science, the best way of predicting a national influenza epidemic is still by the clinical returns of groups of general practitioners co-ordinated through the College's Birmingham Research Unit. Hospital plans, Red Alerts and other forms of health management still depend primarily on the uncorroborated, clinical judgement of practitioners using their eyes, ears and stethoscopes alone.

Yet another approach can be to apply the use of statistics to incidents varying from road deaths to suicide and to other parts of the Health Service, notably hospitals and clinics. All these can now be fed back to practices, to enable them to take an overview of the main needs of their patients.

Clinical effectiveness

A further thrust towards needs assessment has come from the new emphasis on clinical effectiveness. Many traditional treatments are not as effective as patients and doctors would like and outcome measurement argued a quarter of a century ago by Cochrane (1972) remains a clinical challenge.

Despite the biggest gross national product ever recorded in a country still the eighteenth richest in the world, poverty remains a major problem in the UK and a substantial determinant of illness. Wealth still buys health. The Black Report (1980) showed that a baby born into social class 5 had an average expectation of life of 5 years fewer than a baby born in the same city to a social class 1 home. As Watt (1996) has shown, measuring social deprivation is still a powerful predictor not just of illness but of death. General practitioners work face to face with all social classes and are the only clinicians who visit their homes day and night and see first hand the practical impact of living styles and illness.

Occasional Paper 73, Needs Assessment in General Practice has the great advantage of being co-authored by both a consultant in public health medicine who has had a generalist training and a general practitioner. This is not a new subject, nor is it an easy one, but this *Occasional Paper* does provide an overview and introduces a systematic and logical way of thinking about this growing feature of modern primary care. If indeed the future is primary care as encapsulated in the title of the Secretary of State's recent (1996) publication, *Primary Care: The Future*, then it can be certain that these ideas and these techniques will need much more thought in the future. The implications for more rigorous training particularly in numerical and epidemiological skills are obvious and the urgent need for general practice to find a training programme longer than the conventional year will be aided by this development.

Needs Assessment in General Practice can be recommended as the first *Occasional Paper* on this subject. It is unlikely to be the last.

Denis Pereira Gray
Honorary Editor
College Publications

July 1996

References

Black D (Chairman) (1980) *Inequalities in Health*. London, Department of Health and Social Security.

Cochrane A (1972) *Effectiveness and Efficiency*. London, Nuffield Provincial Hospitals Trust.

Eimerl TS (1960) Organised curiosity. *Journal of the Royal College of General Practitioners* **3**, 246–52.

Pereira Gray D, Steele R, Sweeney K et al. (1994) Generalists in medicine. Editorial. *British Medical Journal* **308**, 486–7.

Secretary of State (1989) *Working for Patients*. London, HMSO.

Secretary of State for Health (1996) *Primary Care: The Future*. London, NHS Executive.

Watt GCM (1996) All together now: why social deprivation matters to everyone. *British Medical Journal* **312**, 1026–9.

Watts CAH (1958) How to compile an age-sex register. *Between Ourselves* No.8, 1–12.

Preface

THE NHS reforms of the last few years have changed the face of British general practice. Needs assessment forms the basis of the planning process. Increasing numbers of general practitioners are involved to varying degrees in the commissioning of care. New skills are required to underpin this role. Those engaged in purchasing require locally sensitive information and skills in the assessment of health needs of practice populations.

This guide provides a practical introduction to the topic. The first chapter considers some of the forces shaping general practice today. The second chapter approaches the concept of need from theoretical perspectives. The definition of need as the ability to benefit from health care places particular emphasis on evidence for the effectiveness of that care. New technologies are hastening access to the findings of evaluative research. Critical appraisal skills are now a core part of the doctor's armamentarium. However, effectiveness is only one of several criteria against which planning decisions are made.

Different approaches are outlined in Chapter 3 under four headings. While primary health care teams may want to begin with information they hold, much relevant data are available outside the practice. A particular emphasis is placed on approaches to defining patients' views on health needs.

The following chapter illustrates different approaches in practice. The approaches are complementary. The key to successful health needs analysis lies in reconciling different sources of data. Comprehensive assessment brings together both qualitative and quantitative data. An awareness of the limitations of different data sources is important. The case studies are chosen to demonstrate different issues faced in practice. They illustrate the close relationship of needs assessment to practice profiling, evaluation, audit and even research. Any attempts to summarize a fast-growing literature cannot be wholly comprehensive. Much work in this field goes unpublished and it is hoped this document will prompt further sharing of experience. In the final chapter, a composite approach is outlined.

There is a glossary at the back, which defines the terms used in this *Occasional Paper*.

The justification for dedicating precious time and resources to needs assessment is its impact on subsequent decision-making: does it lead to changes that benefit patients? The reification of needs assessment divorced from other elements of the planning cycle is unhelpful. Practice teams need to know how to use the information at their disposal to develop their own services. A combination of quantitative and qualitative approaches are likely to be most powerful. However, it is through helping to channel resources without the surgery or indeed without the health service—through direct dialogue with their communities—that primary health care professionals may have most scope to effect change.

SJG
SAM

Acknowledgements

The authors would like to thank the following for their ideas, comments and criticisms: John Howie, Julian Tudor Hart, Diane Plamping, Tony Jewell, Graham Buckley and Roger Chapman. In particular, they would like to thank the many people whose work is rudely summarized in Chapter 4 and Vivine Hamilton and Maureen Kerr for their patient secretarial support through numerous drafts of the document.

CHAPTER 1

Background

TRADITIONALLY, general practitioners and public health doctors have sought health goals by different means. General practice has concentrated on personal, continuing health care via the consultation while public health physicians have focused on the population through changes in the environment, society and health service provision (Bhopal, 1995). Various changes are re-aligning these two branches of medical practice. The growth of primary health care teams to encompass community nursing staff, the broadening of the health promotion role in general practice, the increasing involvement of a wider range of professionals in health service planning and policy making are changing the relationship. This chapter reviews the shift of public health work to general practice. New skills are required in primary health care teams to handle these new responsibilities.

Population-oriented primary care

In his thoughtful analysis of what constitutes good general practice, Toon (1994) defines three main models: the biomedical model with its basis in scientific medicine was a product of the Enlightenment; a humanist model, of which the Balint movement is an example, expresses an older philosophical tradition; and a preventive public health model provides a third set of assumptions.

Several authors over the last twenty years have called for the integration of public and primary health care (Russell, 1988). Most have sought to varying extents the wholesale transfer of public health functions into general practice (Hannay, 1993). Less radical commentators have argued that public health doctors should be providing a support function for general practitioners.

Julian Tudor Hart's studies of hypertension from Glyncorrwg provide notable examples of community-oriented general practice (Hart, 1990a). His practice located in a Welsh mining village took responsibility for both community and clinical functions. He stressed the need for accountability to the population served through such means as patient committees, annual reports and meetings (Hart, 1988). He has argued for the need to look in a new way at the relationship between doctors and patients as "co-producers of health" and develop alliances between health workers and the public in defence of health. Tudor Hart's vision was of general practitioners as local community physicians.

Mant and Anderson (1985) proposed that general practitioners accept responsibility for auditing the state of health of their patients, publicizing the results, monitoring and controlling environmentally determined disease, auditing the effectiveness of preventive programmes, and evaluating the effect of medical interventions. Responsibility for these functions has traditionally been vested with public health specialists. Mant and Anderson proposed that these functions be assumed by general practitioners with appropriate transfer of resources to primary care.

Contemporary proponents of an anticipatory care model include the Oxford group, whose writing had a major bearing on the 1990 contract (Fullard et al., 1987). A more community-oriented example is "Healthy Eastenders", a project involving a number of practices in Tower Hamlets (Robson and Falshaw, 1995).

The role of the 'community general practitioner'—a new type of physician who is engaged in local participatory democracy in the pursuit of the maximization of health—remains a minority aspiration but recent changes in the NHS have compelled general practitioners to re-examine their public health role. Anticipatory care with communities may be more cost-effective than with individuals. Whether a general practitioner would be more effective than other public health structures is unknown.

Public health redefined

Public health has been defined as "the science and art of preventing disease, prolonging life and promoting health through the organized efforts of society" (Acheson, 1988). As such it is a function, rather than an area or discipline. The existence of a group of professional workers designated as public health doctors, public health nurses and others including environmental health officers, is an important part of a strategic approach to protecting the health of the populations, but their work is indivisible from that of many other professionals whose activities impact on public health. Primary care professionals are of particular importance.

In Europe and North America, three distinct phases of public health can be identified over the past 150 years (Berridge, 1991). In the nineteenth century the main causes of premature death were infectious diseases accruing against a backcloth of urbanization, poverty and squalor. The Victorian public health movement built on the work of medical officers of health backed up by public health legislation concerning standards for housing and the quality of air, water and food. As the most pressing environmental problems were brought under control, action to improve the health of populations moved on first to personal preventive medical services such as immunization and family planning, and then to a later therapeutic phase (Ashton, 1990).

The beginning of the therapeutic era coincided with the apparent demise of infectious disease and the development of organized treatment services in developed countries (Kickbusch, 1986). Historically, it marked a weakening of departments of public health and of the position of general practitioners and a shift of power and resources to hospital-based medical services. For the next forty years, future improvements in health were thought likely to depend on further technological advances.

This medical scientific domination was increasingly challenged by the early 1970s. Most countries were experiencing a crisis in health care funding irrespective of the structure of their health services or the methods of financing them. This escalation in costs was in part a consequence of technological innovation in treatment methods and in part a consequence of major demographic changes with the growth of elderly populations. Critiques of the domination of secondary and tertiary care reflected these wider political and economic imperatives (Illich, 1975; McKeown, 1976).

The Lalonde Report in 1974 inaugurated a new era of public health by focusing attention on the fact that much premature death and disability was preventable. What is often called the "new public health" is a synthesis of environmental and lifestyle change together with appropriate medical interventions (Ashton and Seymour, 1988). Many contemporary health problems—mental, cardiovascular, cancers, and age-related—have social antecedents which require health protective public policies.

The Alma-Ata declaration stressed community participation, intersectoral action and the reorientation of medical care towards health promotion, prevention and primary medical care as prerequisites for implementation of WHO strategy (WHO, 1978). This reorientation involved a shift from primary medical care (a professional concept based on teams of health workers in the community) to primary health care (a social concept concerned with populations as well as individuals). Primary health care was seen as the means through which the public health function could best be implemented (WHO, 1981).

Less grandiose considerations have drawn public health practitioners back from the periphery of medical practice. The power of medical officers declined with the creation of the NHS in 1948 and was further reduced following the NHS reorganization of 1974. The specialty of community medicine fell into abeyance. However, the NHS reforms reversed this. They placed new responsibilities on health authorities for the assessment of their populations' health needs (NHSME, 1991). Particular skills were required. Notwithstanding concerns that public health practitioners might be compromised addressing a managerial agenda (Whitty and Jones, 1992), the specialty has been reinvigorated over the last six years.

Bridging the divide

At the heart of the relationship between general practice and public health is an ethical conflict between individual and collective freedom. The enduring strength of general practice is its concern with the 'individual in context'. This bond is hallowed in the consultation. The clinical generalist develops a unique understanding of the social, spiritual and environmental determinants of their patients' health. The utilitarian values underpinning population-oriented care are at odds with the individualistic nature of the traditional doctor-patient relationship. However, the roles of carer, advocate and enabler may overlap and conflict with one another. Traditional primary care based on the perspective of the clinician exposed exclusively to individual patients presenting for care has evident limitations. There are several reasons why a population focus in clinical care is desirable.

First, knowledge about the distribution of health problems in the community cannot be derived from experience in the practice alone. Most episodes of ill health do not lead to a medical consultation (White et al., 1961).

Secondly, knowledge of how disease presents is not obtainable without a population focus. Thirdly, doctors overestimate their role in the provision of care (Helman, 1984). Primary health care is not, of course, synonymous with general practice and is provided through a range of other people in the community. Most of what is known about illness and its management derives from patients' encounters in treatment centres. Professional knowledge about disease does not necessarily reflect people's illness experiences and needs to be supplemented with the insights of the community (Blaxter, 1995).

Several international trends in the delivery of health services are facilitating community-oriented approaches to primary care (Rogers, 1982). Financial remuneration for practice in primary care has improved more than that for the practice of sub-specialty medicine in many parts of the world (Hsiao et al., 1988). Secondly, the physician is no longer the sole 'captain of the ship'. As patients survive longer and the burdens of morbidity increase in community settings, other health personnel become increasingly central to the maintenance of well-being. Thirdly, attention is being given to the need to make training programmes for doctors more relevant to changing population needs. In the UK, undergraduate curricula are being radically reappraised (Oswald, 1989). The theoretical (pre-clinical) and practical (clinical) components of medical training are being reintegrated (GMC, 1993). More training is now taking place in community settings (Murray and Modell, 1995). Fourthly, an emphasis on more effective and more efficient health care will promote community-oriented approaches if they prevent disease and encourage more discriminating use of medical technologies. Primary health care teams have always been pivotally placed to combine high risk and population approaches to disease prevention (Rose, 1992).

In seeking to reconcile primary health care and public health, a balance must be found between the integrative approaches of person-centred care and the reductionism of the population perspective. The next challenge is to identify the skills and functions which are needed to address the tasks in hand and to plan the education, training and research to support them.

Primary care led purchasing

Several issues placed reform in general practice high on the political agenda by the late 1980s (Day, 1992). Spending on primary health care was growing at a faster rate than expenditure on hospital and community services. Expenditure on prescribing in particular was demand led and could not be kept under control. In addition, there were anxieties about the state of general practice in the inner cities (Acheson, 1981). There was growing interest in prevention and the role that general practitioners might play in this.

The white paper *Promoting Better Health* (Secretary of State, 1987) laid the foundations for a new GP contract (DoH and Welsh Office, 1989). The proposals were intended to achieve three main policy aims: to improve the quality of general practice, to make professional providers more sensitive to consumer preferences, and to bring greater managerial control over the activities of general practitioners, in particular their prescribing.

Working for Patients concentrated on increasing efficiency by introducing an 'internal market' through which health care purchasing was to be separated from service provision (Secretary of State, 1989). Whereas district health authorities were exhorted to carry out formal needs assessments as the basis for their purchasing plans and to balance priorities for the complete range of health care needs in a large population, general practitioner fundholders were expected to respond to their patients' demands by purchasing a selected range of services for relatively small practice populations.

The third major tranche of government reforms were laid down in the white paper *Caring for People* (DoH et al., 1990). This heralded the introduction of a comparable purchaser/provider split in the social services departments of local authorities. Its impact on the working lives of general practitioners who play a major part in the assessment of individuals' health and social care needs may indirectly be as large as the other changes described (Kingdom and Sumners, 1995). In many parts of the country, primary health care teams are establishing closer links with local social workers. The care managers purchasing social care are aligned to do so on behalf of groups of practices. In some places, this brings closer the prospect of genuine joint commissioning.

The introduction of fundholding was seen as the 'wild card' in the pack of reforms. Despite early opposition, the scheme has gained favour with many general practitioners and now covers over 50% of the population (Ham and Shapiro, 1995).

Fundholding has been widely hailed by politicians and participants as a success. Fundholders have undoubtedly proved agile as purchasers extracting new services and quality standards from service providers (Glennerster et al., 1994). Many of these achievements have indirectly benefited non-fundholders. However, the evidence that fundholding has improved the quality of care or of communication between general practitioners and hospital consultants remains limited (Coulter, 1992; Newton et al., 1993; Le Grand, 1994; Howie et al., 1994, 1995). There is little evidence that fundholders' purchasing plans have been based on systematic assessments of their populations' needs (Audit Commission, 1996). The transaction costs incurred in dealing with numerous small-scale purchasers are greater than when purchasing is carried out by one district health authority (Dixon and Glennerster, 1995). Whether the greater cost of this form of purchasing is justified in terms of greater health benefits is unknown (Coulter, 1995). Budget-setting for fundholders remains problematic (Dixon, 1994). Budgets are still based largely on past patterns of service use and have varied widely (Day and Klein, 1991; Dixon et al., 1994). The Department of Health has been anxious to move towards capitation-based funding but the construction of a robust weighted formula for populations of 5000 is prob-

ably impossible (Sheldon et al., 1994). The constraints small denominators place on needs assessment will be discussed again in Chapter 3.

Despite the lack of evidence of benefit and despite obvious risks, in September 1994 the Secretary of State for Health announced her intention to extend fundholding to smaller practices (NHSE, 1994). This marked a significant shift towards demand-led purchasing away from a system with an allocation based on historical usage.

In addition to standard fundholding, two new models have been offered to entice the undecided. Practices entering community fundholding (or 'primary care purchasing' in Scotland) can purchase their own staff, computers and a limited range of community services. Most political interest has focused on total fundholding where practices—singly or in groups—are purchasing an expanded range of services for larger populations.

Health authorities are supposed to be developing many of their purchasing functions. Their skills and resources are to support increasing numbers of general practitioners in the business of needs assessment and contracting. Newly fused district health authorities, family health services authorities and health boards are to develop strategy and monitor providers' performance in the light of those strategies. These bodies will struggle to support an increasing diversity of small-scale purchasers. Numerous alternative commissioning models, many based on localities, are evolving (Ham, 1993; Black et al., 1994; Graffy and Williams, 1994; Shapiro, 1994).

Whatever the future for particular models, the principles underlying 'primary care led purchasing'—the bringing of decision-making as close to the patient as possible, the devolution of budgetary responsibility, strengthening the hand of the general practitioner as co-ordinator of care—seem set to endure. The skills that underpin effective and equitable commissioning need to be developed rapidly in primary health care teams. These skills include an understanding of data sources and their limitations, competencies in needs analysis, and service evaluation.

Summary

There is a long tradition of attempts to fuse the practice of community medicine and primary medical care. *Working for Patients* inaugurated the most radical changes in the NHS since its inception but reinforced policies underpinning the new general practitioner contract. The balance of power within the medical profession has swung markedly in favour of general practitioners but with new powers have come new responsibilities. Increasing numbers of general practitioners are involved to varying degrees in the commissioning of care. New skills are required to underpin this role. Those engaged in purchasing require locally sensitive information and skills in the assessment of health needs.

CHAPTER 2
Theoretical perspectives

The nature of need

PRIMARY health care teams spend much time assessing the needs of individuals; many know less about defining the needs of a practice population. The need for health underlies but does not wholly determine the need for health care (Gillam, 1992a). Health care needs are often measured in terms of demand, but demand is to a great extent 'supply-induced'. For example, variations in practice referral or consultation rates have less to do with the health status of the populations served than with differences between doctors, such as their skills or referral thresholds (Saunders et al., 1989).

There is no generally accepted definition of 'need'. Last's notion of the 'clinical iceberg' of disease (Last, 1963) has been supported by various community studies indicating much illness unknown to health professionals. Needs can be classified in terms of diseases, priority groups, geographical areas, services or using a lifecycle approach (children/teenagers/adults/elderly). The literature available to inform needs assessment is limited. Few interventions have been fully evaluated. Many beneficial outcomes are emotional or subjective in nature and difficult to quantify (Metcalfe, 1990). Few outcome measures have been validated for use in primary care settings (Wilkin et al., 1992).

Bradshaw's taxonomy of need is perhaps the most frequently quoted analysis (Bradshaw, 1972). It highlights four types of need:

- Expressed needs (needs expressed by action, for instance visiting a doctor)

- Normative needs (defined by experts)

- Comparative needs (comparing one group of people with another)

- Felt needs (those needs people say they have).

The variety of approaches to needs assessment reflect the variety of professionals involved and changing historical concerns (Stevens and Gabbay, 1991). The public health model currently predominant in the Department of Health seeks to integrate these different perspectives. Needs are defined in terms of the population's ability to benefit from health care (NHSME, 1991). The following five distinctions are worth emphasizing:

Health or health care?

Health is famously difficult to define. The World Health Organization's definition of health embraces the physical, social, and emotional well-being of an individual, group, or community and emphasizes health as a positive resource of life, not just the absence of disease (WHO, 1978). Health needs accordingly encompass education, social services, housing, the environment and social policy.

The need for health care is the population's ability to benefit from health care which is in turn the sum of many individuals' ability to benefit (Matthew, 1972; Culyer, 1976). In the past, this has only been assessed on the basis of epidemiological research rather than clinical records. However, increasing computerization in general practice provides the basis for much more detailed local study in future (Shanks et al., 1995).

As well as treatment, health care includes prevention, diagnosis, continuing care, rehabilitation and palliative care. The ability to benefit does not mean that all outcomes will be favourable but implies benefits that will on average be effective. Some benefits may be manifested in changes of clinical status; others such as the benefits of reassurance or the support of carers are difficult to measure. Diagnosis and reassurance form an important part of primary care when many people may require no more than a negative diagnosis (Stevens and Raftery, 1993). Health care needs assessment thus requires knowledge of the incidence of the health problem (risk factor, disease, disability), its prevalence, and the effectiveness of services to address them.

Individual or population?

Clinicians focus on the individual with need defined in terms of what can be done for the patient consulting. However, this may neglect the health needs of people not attending surgery. Traditionally, the clinical view enshrined in such notions as 'clinical freedom' has taken little account of treatment cost. Services of doubtful efficacy are provided if they may be even remotely beneficial to patients. In contrast, the public health view seeks to prioritize within finite budgets. Individual clinical decisions may be made without considering the opportunity costs of treatment, while at a population level such opportunity costs must be minimized if the health of the population is to be maximized (Williams, 1989).

The ethical conflicts raised are not easily resolved. Health professionals will only reluctantly withhold interventions of minor benefit for the greater good of potential patients. Tension between what is best for the individual and what may be best for society will always present a dilemma for clinicians. In reality, a complex range of considerations of which cost-effectiveness is but one will always determine both clinical and strategic decision-making.

Need, supply or demand?

Health care is never organized as a 'pure' market. Its products are heavily subsidized and regulated in all countries (Williams, 1976). The main reasons for this is asymmetry of information whereby patients lack knowledge of their own treatment needs and depend on providers to make appropriate decisions (Mooney, 1986). The doctor acts as the patient's 'agent' to translate demands into needs. However, the literature on variation in referrals, prescribing, and other activity rates reveals that this agency relationship is complex (Wennberg et al., 1988).

Professional perceptions of need may differ from those of consumers (Bowling et al., 1993). The latter are more likely to be influenced by external factors such as media coverage and the opinions of relatives and friends. Consumers' priorities vary with age, health status and previous experience of health service use (Blaxter, 1995; Bowling, 1996).

The health problems considered to constitute need may change over time. Much universal screening activity, for example in the field of child health surveillance, is no longer supported by research evidence (Butler, 1989; Hall, 1992). New needs accrue with the development of new technology. There is usually a time lag before lay demand (for health) reflects scientific evidence of need (for health care). Unfortunately, an even longer time lag distorts the provision of health services. Their supply is affected by historical factors, and by public and political pressures. The closure of hospital beds is ever politically charged. Health services tend to be regarded as untouchable even when their usefulness has been outlived, while medical innovations are generally implemented before they have been fully evaluated.

Stevens and Gabbay (1991) have usefully illustrated the relationship between need, demand and supply. Figure 1 shows seven fields of services divided into those for which there is a need but no demand or supply (1), those for which there is a demand but no need or supply (2), those for which there is a supply but no need or demand (3), and various other degrees of overlap. Any intervention can be fitted into one of these fields. Rehabilitation after myocardial infarction may be needed but not supplied or demanded. Antibiotics for upper respiratory tract infection may be demanded but not needed or supplied, and so on. Much effort is required on behalf of patients, providers and purchasers to make the three cycles more confluent. Something is known about how to change professional behaviour through financial incentives, protocols, education, audit and even contracts: the factors influencing patient preferences are less well understood.

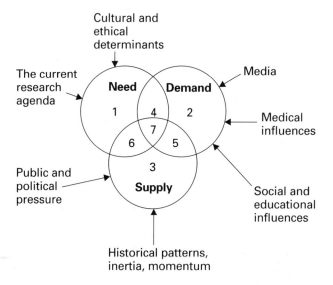

Figure 1 Need, demand and supply (Stevens and Gabbay, 1991). Reproduced with permission.

Practice needs or population needs?

In beginning to identify health care needs, it is easy to confuse the needs of the practice team with those of the practice's patients. Needs can be considered in geographical terms (for example, the most deprived estate in the catchment area) or in terms of priority groups (for example, the high proportion of ethnic minorities on the practice list). Health needs, especially in relation to community services, blur easily into demands for more staff. The need for more care for children at risk, for example, does not necessarily equate with a need for more health visitors. In this example, the same staff may more effectively divide their time or other key personnel may address the need. It is important to be explicit about these distinctions if health needs assessment is not to veil unquestioning demands for more staff, training, practice computers or resources that cannot automatically be assumed to benefit patients.

Practice population or community?

Much demographic, census and public health information is collected and analysed at ward level. It relates to geographical areas. Practice populations are often spread across several wards particularly in urban areas. On one Edinburgh housing estate, residents were registered with 43 different practices (Murray et al., 1995). This creates problems for those seeking to utilize census and other ward-based information. It is possible using post codes to map these data and derive weighted census variables but the resources to undertake this are in short supply.

The planning cycle

The planning cycle should originate in an assessment of needs: where are we now and where do we want to get to? The rest of the cycle is mostly concerned with how to get there (Figure 2). Comprehensive needs assessment will generate a bewildering array of possible needs. There are many ways of identifying priorities. These often involve a form of ranking. The use of a decision matrix is illustrated in Chapter 4. Various criteria may be used in ranking priorities. They include size of the health problem (prevalence and incidence), its severity in terms of morbidity or mortality, the availability of effective interventions, the feasibility of the work entailed for the primary

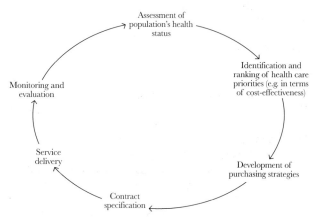

Figure 2 Planning cycle

health care team, the level of group interest, and the costs and resources required.

The prioritizing process should involve as many of the team who will be affected by the choice as reasonably possible. Teams need to take careful stock of their current work when making a decision. In many important areas work may already be ongoing (for example, heart disease prevention). Few health professionals are not already overloaded. There is little point in setting grandiose objectives that cannot realistically be attained.

Audit and evaluation (to see whether we have got to where we want to go) is therefore integrally related to needs assessment. Indeed, the selection of audit topics should be framed by systematic assessment of priority needs. It is usually governed by ad hoc medical choices.

Descriptions of the planning process falsely imply an orderly sequence. Few general practitioners with much experience of planning and policy-making will subscribe to this myth of rational planning. In real life, it is rarely possible to maintain forward progress around the cycle for long. The process is iterative rather than cyclical. The commonest causes of disruption, other than shortage of finance, are vague objectives, lack of information and changing circumstances, people and politics. An understanding of the contingent nature of much planning is important in effecting change. Implementation is discussed further in Chapter 5.

Evidence-based practice

The internal market has focused attention as never before on the effectiveness of health care. It has been claimed that fewer than a quarter of health care interventions have been fully evaluated (Eddy, 1991). This underestimates the extent to which routine general practice is evidence based (Gill et al., 1996) but needs assessment exposes deficiencies in our knowledge base. Screening for cystic fibrosis, minimally invasive surgery and near patient testing in general practice provide recent examples of areas where new technologies are being diffused before full evaluation. The pressure to optimize value for money from finite purchasing budgets has focused particular attention on the primary/secondary care interface.

Producing the evidence is the main task of the NHS Research and Development initiative (DoH, 1993a). The recent development of robust methods for undertaking systematic reviews should provide the knowledge on which evidence-based practice can be founded. Until recently, there have been few mechanisms within the National Health Service to promote the implementation of research findings.

The development of a national research strategy is a major step forward, but there is frequently an unacceptable delay between evidence of effectiveness of a specific intervention appearing in medical literature and change in clinical practice (NHSME, 1993a). Explanations include the sheer volume of literature and the inability of many health professionals to appraise critically the information about effectiveness that is presented to them.

Four main strategies for promoting evidence-based practice have been proposed: patient-centred, educational, administrative and economic (Haines and Jones, 1994). Patient-centred approaches include educating patients about the effectiveness of interventions in an attempt to change the behaviour of professionals and patients. Educational approaches that are likely to be effective incorporate feedback of performance, involvement of learners in setting priorities, and educational activities that are linked closely to clinical practice. Administrative approaches include clinical audit and management structures to promote evidence-based practice. Economic strategies are frequently motivated by the intention to contain costs but may be used to promote clinical effectiveness.

Although comparatively little research has been undertaken to determine the most effective strategies for promoting evidence-based practice, systematic reviews have suggested that guidelines, continuing education, audit, feedback and computerized decision support systems may all be effective in some circumstances. This has led to a rapid expansion (where possible) of evidence-based clinical guidelines (Grimshaw and Russell, 1993). Their more naïve proponents see these as the solution to controlling bad doctors, inappropriate health care, spiralling NHS costs and the rationing dilemma. It is argued that, if ineffective practices are abandoned, then sufficient resources will be released for those procedures of demonstrable value (Hunter, 1994).

Increasingly, it is necessary to build up an integrated system to promote evidence-based practice that links research and development with education and clinical audit. Five key groups need to be considered in developing an integrated strategy for implementation: purchasers, providers, professional organizations and educational bodies, patients and policy makers. The strategy to promote evidence-based practice cannot be seen merely as a central initiative but must actively involve those whose practice needs to be continually updated (Taylor, 1996). However, zealotry in the cause of 'EBM' needs to be tempered. An extreme rationalistic emphasis on randomized controlled trials as the gold standard can distort priority setting in areas such as mental health and primary care that may always be less amenable to these methods. Appropriate observational methods should not be devalued (Black, 1996).

Appraising evidence

General practitioners glean new information from many sources. These include summaries from the medical literature (reviews, practice guidelines, consensus statements, editorials and summaries of articles in 'throwaway' publications); consultations with colleagues who have special expertise; lectures; seminars; advertisements in medical journals; conversations with representatives from pharmaceutical companies; and original articles in journals and journal supplements. Each of these sources is subject to its own particular biases (Rennie and Bero, 1990; Bero et al., 1992). Clinicians need ways of systematically filtering this welter of information. The same skills are required for health needs assessment.

The first step is to frame clinical questions that are pertinent and answerable. Thus, for example, to answer the question: "Do males in my practice need to be screened for prostate cancer?", the question might be: "What is the evidence that screening symptomless males using prostate-specific antigen testing reduces their risk of dying from prostate cancer?''

The next step is to track down the relevant literature. The ability to conduct electronic searches of the medical literature is fast becoming a basic skill in modern practice. Textbooks are at least partly out of date before they are published. Though frequent updates help, they do not ensure that their conclusions are valid. Most books and review articles do not qualify as scientific reviews (Mulrow, 1987). Electronic access to Medline is readily available in a variety of on-line and CD-ROM formats. The addition of structured abstracts to Medline and the development of databases that have screened articles for their validity and clinical relevance such as the Cochrane databases and the electronic version of the ACP journal club (see Appendix 1) promise to make the task of retrieving information from the medical literature even easier.

The third step is to decide whether the article—usually a literature review—is likely to provide valid results that will help. The user guides to the medical literature developed by the McMaster Group (Oxman et al., 1994) are a valuable starting point. These have provided the basis for the CASP programme promoted from the Institute of Health Sciences in Oxford (Milne, 1995). The 10 questions shown in Table 1 help make sense of the evidence. If the answers to the first two screening questions are negative, it is probably not worth proceeding with the rest.

Table 1 Critical appraisal—the questions

A. Are the results of the review valid?

Screening questions

1. *Did the review address a clearly focused issue?*
   An issue can be 'focused' in terms of:
   - the population studied
   - the intervention given
   - the outcomes considered

2. *Did the authors select the right sort of studies for the review?*
   The 'right sort of studies' would:
   - address the review's question
   - have an adequate study design

Detailed questions

3. *Do you think the important, relevant studies were included?*
   Look for:
   - which bibliographic databases were used
   - checks from reference lists
   - personal contact with experts
   - unpublished as well as published studies
   - non-English language studies

4. *Did the review's authors do enough to assess the quality of the included studies?*
   The authors need to consider the rigour of the studies they have identified. Lack of rigour may affect the studies' results. (All that glistens is not gold!)

5. *Were the results similar from study to study?*
   Consider whether:
   - the results of all the included studies are clearly displayed

- the results of the different studies are similar
- the reasons for any variations in results are discussed

B. What are the results?

6. *What is the overall result of the review?*
   Consider:
   - if you are clear about the review's 'bottom line' results
   - what these are (numerically if appropriate)
   - what units these results are expressed in

7. *How precise are the results?*
   Are there confidence limits? What are they?

C. Will the results help locally?

8. *Can the results be applied to the local population?*
   Do you think that the patients covered by the review are similar enough to your population?

9. *Were all clinically important outcomes considered?*
   If not, does this affect the decision?

10. *Are the benefits worth the harms and costs?*
    This is unlikely to be addressed by the review. But what do you think?

Sources of data

The sources of information required to support health care needs assessment lie at different levels (Figure 3). The most important, of course, is the practice population. The views of patients on needs and services to meet those needs can be gleaned directly in various ways (page 10). Other sources of data can be divided into those internal and those external to the practice.

Sources within the practice include the practice computer, community nursing records, audit reports and PACT data (see Chapter 3). Access to the many external sources of data can be gained via the local district department of public health or a well-equipped medical library. Key

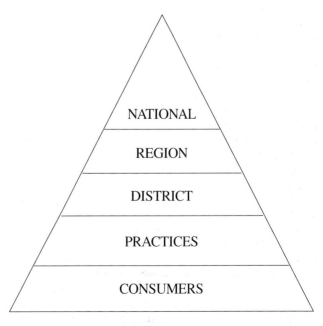

Figure 3 Information tiers

public health data are listed in Table 2. A fuller description of these data items is given in Appendix 2. The results of local and national surveys, census data and research are compiled at district level. Most DHA departments of public health and medical libraries can provide access to the 'grey' literature or key databases. Many are nowadays equipped with CD-ROM and the Internet access that are transforming other areas of medical practice. Time and effort invested in personal contact with local librarians and in mastering these technologies will yield big dividends.

Table 2 Summary of public health data

Demographic data	Source
Estimated present population	OPCS population estimates
Five-year population projections	OPCS population projections by age bands
Social characteristics	Census, Labour Force Survey
Deprivation, Jarman	Health authorities/health boards
Housing	National Dwelling Survey ACORN, Regional Council
Activity data	
Process data, hospital	Korner data, KO forms, RHAs in England (Korner Aggregated Returns System: KARS), KES (Korner Episode Statistics) data
Process data, community	Scottish Morbidity Records in Scotland. Korner data, KC, KT forms
Hospitalization rates	Department of Health PIs, Regions
Performance indicators	Department of Health
Health data	
Data relating to births	*OPCS Monitor VS1*
Perinatal mortality rates	*OPCS Monitor VS1*
Infant mortality rates	*OPCS Monitor VS1*
Abortions	*OPCS Monitor AB*
Deaths by selected causes	*OPCS Monitor VS3*
Standardized mortality rates for selected cause of death	Regions
Infectious diseases	*OPCS Monitors MB, WR*
Morbidity	*General Household Survey,* Royal College of General Practitioners Morbidity Survey, GP consolidated computer networks (e.g. GPASS in Scotland)

Health authorities have access to much comparative activity data that underpin their 'pay and rations' functions. Care needs to be taken in sharing potentially sensitive information but too little use is made of these data for planning purposes.

Summary

In this chapter the concept of need has been examined. The definition of need as the ability to benefit from health care places a particular emphasis on evidence for the effectiveness of that care. However, effectiveness is only one of several criteria against which planning decisions are made.

The results of health technology assessment constantly redefine doctors' perceptions of what their patients need. The developing science of systematic reviews and new initiatives such as the Cochrane Collaboration will hasten access to the findings of evaluative research. Critical appraisal skills may be as integral to good doctoring in future as clinical or management skills are today.

CHAPTER 3
Approaches to needs assessment

Approaches to needs assessment can be categorized in different ways. The classification chosen here parallels Bradshaw's taxonomy of need. Approaches are considered under four headings described below.

1. Practice-defined approach

The primary health care team is ideally placed to assess the health needs of its registered population. Members of the team typically have contact with 70% of registered patients annually and 90% of all health problems are dealt with in the primary care setting (Fry, 1993). An advantage of needs assessment at practice level is that solutions to problems can often be found more easily when supported by detailed local knowledge and research (NHS Training Division, 1994). However, just as general practitioners frequently fail to recognize individual needs in the community (Reid, 1992; Hopton and Dlugolecka, 1995), an undisciplined eye may neglect the needs of particular sections of a practice population. In Bradshaw's terms, this approach reflects expressed needs—or demands.

As important as all other sources of data on the practice population is the collective knowledge of the practice team members themselves. The knowledge of those on the ground is often derided as 'anecdotal'. The product of many years' direct experience of working in the neighbourhood, this intimate local knowledge is frequently the richest of sources. It is important to be as systematic as possible in the collection of these data. All practice team members can contribute to this process. This is unlikely to happen where the culture of the practice does not value the unique skills and competencies of different team members. In this respect, the contributions of community nursing staff who may feel themselves to be outside the team are often in danger of being overlooked. Ways of systematizing multidisciplinary input are discussed in Chapter 4. Fellowship by Assessment, a quality assurance programme developed by the Royal College of General Practitioners, describes the practice-based data considered to have greatest utility in assessing and meeting needs (RCGP, 1995).

The health status and health needs of a population can be assessed using information from the practice register, the health visiting profile, and other primary health care team resources (Schofield, 1992; see page 15). The Health Visitors Association advocates the drawing up of practice profiles as fundamental to developing a pro-active approach to primary care (Twinn et al., 1992). The Royal College of Nursing (1993) has also suggested a structure for the 'practice population profile'.

There are simple direct measures of socio-economic status that can be collected routinely by practices (such as car or house ownership) to help target needs created by persisting social inequalities in health (Hopton et al., 1992).

Hart et al. (1991) have described case finding and audit in a socially deprived community (see page 15).

Anticipatory care is possible if practices are highly motivated with sufficient resources, trained staff, appropriate organization and a targeted approach based on research. Otherwise Hart considers that the 'rule of halves' (Smith et al., 1990) will continue to apply: half of all specific health needs are not known, half of those known are not helped, and half the help is not effective.

What has been described as 'living epidemiology' (Gray et al., 1994) can start with routine data extracted from age-sex and morbidity registers. Practices hold much information (Shanks et al., 1995) but the volume and quality of data vary (Boyle, 1993; Wilson et al., 1995) and diverse, qualitative 'soft' material is difficult to analyse. Some practices enter diagnoses and outcomes at each consultation while others record manually only basic information (Chisholm, 1990). The Read codes may overcome the problem that different doctors may use different terms to classify an illness but doctors may diagnose the same symptoms in very different ways. Computer databases in general practice will be useful planning tools only when data of good quality are collected (Pringle and Hobbs, 1991). However, to paraphrase Charles Babbage, inadequate data are better than no data at all providing their limitations are acknowledged.

In Scotland, 75% of the population are registered in 850 practices with a standardized computer software system, GPASS. Completeness and accuracy of this database are improving but morbidity recording is still about 10% short of proxy prescribing rates (Taylor et al., 1993). Data from 11 representative practices in Somerset have been validated for use in support of evidence-based purchasing (Pearson et al., 1996). It is important to remember that what practice databases record is not the morbidity of the practice population but the morbidity that the doctor thinks he or she sees. All patient records reflect the way in which the doctor has organized the illness that is presented to him or her (Marinker, 1967).

Data can be found in books or registers kept in the practice, such as referrals, diagnostic tests, deaths and home visits. Computerized data include chronic illness, repeat prescribing details, and various screening and health promotion data. Approximately 20 patients on an average list of 2000 people die each year. Over time, death registers can provide valuable information for audit (Berlin et al., 1993; Wagstaff et al., 1994). Practice annual reports may be helpful in assessing needs (Record et al., 1994) if standardized data have been collected.

Information that may be available at practice level which can assist health needs assessment is listed in Table 3.

Table 3 Data at practice level

- Prevalence of chronic illness
- Incidence of acute illnesses and symptoms
- Contacts with general practitioners
  —surgery consultation rate/1000 patients/per year
  —house call rate/1000
  —out-of-hours visits/1000

—night visits/1000
—telephone advice/1000
- Contacts with other members of the primary health care team
  —practice nurse
  —health visitor
  —district nurse
  —others
- Prescribing details
  —repeat (from computer register)
  —total prescribing figures (PACT or Scottish prescribing analysis)
- Use of investigations
  —laboratory samples (bacteriology, haematology etc.)
  —radiology
  —ECGs
- Outpatient referrals
  —hospital, by specialty
  —physiotherapy, chiropody, occupational therapy
- Attendance rate at accident and emergency department
- Hospital admissions
- Health promotion and disease prevention data
  —smoking, drinking, drug users, BMI data, immunization coverage levels (2-year-olds and 5-year-olds)
  —cervical cytology
- Death register
  —causes, place of death, preventable factors
- Socio-economic status
  —details of deprivation payments
  —telephone ownership percentage
  —medical records may reveal unemployment, domestic problems
- Knowledge (explicit and implicit of the primary health care team)
  —health visitor: practice profile, breast feeding rates, use of other agencies
  —district nurse: workload details
  —practice nurse: workload details, for example influenza coverage rate (note that a great deal of data from community nurses are forwarded to their managers without informing the primary health care team)
- Other sources
  —suggestions box

2. Comparative approach

The comparative approach to needs assessment contrasts health data and levels of service uptake in one practice population with similar information from other practices locally or nationally. Much practice-based needs assessment and audit have traditionally involved comparative activity analysis. However, difficulties of interpretation abound. The large literature seeking to explain variations in referral rates illustrates these difficulties (Roland and Coulter, 1993). Do low referral rates indicate more comprehensive management in primary care or lower diagnostic competence? The evidence suggests that variations reflect differences in individual referral thresholds rather than differences in patient populations. The range of comparative indicators available at different levels of the service is discussed in Chapter 4. The DoH Health Service Indicators provide valuable information on variation in costs and service provision at district level (DoH, 1993b).

Several global indices are used to assess need in geographical terms. Jarman's Underprivileged Area score remains the most widely used unitary measure of depriva-

tion (Jarman, 1984). Designed as a measure of general practitioners' workload, its validity has been questioned (Davey Smith, 1991).

Routine workload data can be used comparatively to demonstrate inequitable use of services. A study in a Nottingham practice revealed a 2.8-fold variation in the night visit rate between wards. Much of the variation was explained by the Townsend deprivation score (Carlisle et al., 1993). Various other comparative data can help identify putative practice needs, for example ancillary staffing levels, data on immunization, cervical cytology uptake or PACT (prescribing activity and cost).

Morbidity information may form the basis of comparative analysis at practice level. Having calculated expected prevalences of disease and their sub-categories, the practice may compare these with the figures observed. Differences between observed and expected prevalence rates serve as a starting point. They raise questions. For example, is a lower than expected prevalence of diabetes a function of poor case finding, inadequate recording, or is it attributable to demographic features of the practice population?

The RCGP Birmingham Research Unit collates data from over 90 practices in its decennial morbidity surveys. These provide valuable data for the purposes of comparison (McCormick et al., 1995). Detailed mortality and limited morbidity data are available at district and ward level through the Office of Population Censuses and Surveys (DoH, 1993c). Again, these data often refer to wards rather than practice populations. They may be viewed both as measures of need and as population outcome measures, although health care is not necessarily a major determinant of mortality and morbidity (DoH, 1993c).

3. Epidemiological/public health approach

An epidemiological/public health approach is an example of the normative approach. It is the mainstay of public health practitioners working in health authorities purchasing services for large populations. This approach considers need in terms of diseases rather than population groups or services. Data derived from attested research studies (surveys, effectiveness literature) are applied to the population of the locality or practice. Effectiveness and prevalence studies are often generally applicable but care must be taken where practice populations differ extensively from national norms in terms of age, sex or ethnic breakdown. Local costs also vary widely. The use of measures of cost utility (for example, the Quality Adjusted Life Year) for evaluating interventions requires careful interpretation (Drummond, 1980; Gudex 1986).

Stages of the epidemiologically based approach to needs assessment are as follows:

(a) Defining the problem

All diagnostic labels attached to a particular health problem should be identified, although these can be falsely inclusive (for example, sore throats are sometimes labelled tonsillitis to justify antibiotic prescription). Sub-categories need to be delineated. For example, if the particular concern is postpartum depression, minor episodes of anxiety and depression, chronic psychotic illness and other categories need to be excluded.

(b) Frequency of occurrence

The distinction between prevalence and incidence is fundamental to the understanding of needs assessment (Table 4). High incidence is not synonymous with need for effective management. The incidence of a common cold may say little about the need for general practice consultations. However, with the growing burden of chronic degenerative disease managed in general practice, the prevalence of chronic diseases such as cardiovascular disease, diabetes and asthma is of critical interest.

Table 4: Prevalence/incidence

Incidence rate	=	$\dfrac{\text{Number of new cases in period}}{\text{Number at risk in period}}$
(Point) prevalence rate	=	$\dfrac{\text{Number of persons with the disease at a point in time}}{\text{Total population}}$

(c) Services utilized

Although these may not reflect need, local service levels provide a baseline for comparative analysis (see below). Provision of health care can be difficult to quantify. Most routinely available information concerns health care processes such as patient contacts (in the community) or hospital discharges. Where the process is well defined such as elective surgery (for example, hip or knee replacements), process information is most useful.

(d) Effectiveness and cost-effectiveness of services

A growing emphasis on evidence-based practice is spawning a number of valuable resources for health professionals (Table 5; Appendix 2). A range of different models has evolved for the management of many chronic health problems. Given that need is derived from measures of incidence, prevalence and effectiveness, economic analyses of the most cost-effective service options are increasing (NHSME, 1995). For example, the OXCHECK and British family heart studies have all been submitted to exhaustive economic analysis (Field et al., 1995; Langham et al., 1996; Wonderling et al., 1996).

Table 5 Sources of effectiveness information

Institutions
- NHS Centre for Reviews and Dissemination
- UK Health Outcomes Clearing House

Documents which will be useful in carrying out macro-level reviews of services
- Health Needs Assessment Documents
- *Health of the Nation* Key Area Handbooks

Documents which will be useful for reviewing the detailed provision of services
- *Effective Health Care Bulletins*
- Cochrane Databases
- Confidential Enquiry Reports (Stillbirths and Deaths in Infancy, Maternal Deaths, Perioperative and Operative Deaths, and Counselling for Genetic Disorders)
- Consultation Documents on Health Outcome Indicators
- *Health of the Nation* Target Effectiveness Documents

However, for most conditions the information available on disease incidence/prevalence, cost-effectiveness or thresholds for intervention is inadequate.

4. Patient-defined approach

A patient-defined approach to needs assessment is based on the demands, wishes and different perspectives of people on the practice list. The NHS reforms were supposed to promote greater responsiveness to users. The growth in consumerism as reflected in Patient's Charter initiatives, attempts to render fundholders accountable, and the development of audit are further encouraging the direct involvement of patients (Neve and Taylor, 1995). There are many ways of engaging patients in priority setting. Patient feedback can be obtained from suggestion boxes, participation groups, public meetings, interviews and postal surveys.

Qualitative strategies

Qualitative methods involve listening to people and becoming involved in their world—an exciting process that is already a motivating force for some general practitioners (Britten and Fisher, 1993). Qualitative research encompasses a variety of methods such as semi-structured interviewing, observational studies, group discussions, and the analysis of written documents. Qualitative research can close the gap between the sciences of discovery and implementation (Jones, 1995). A range of qualitative techniques is needed to complement quantitative research (Pope and Mays, 1995). They are especially relevant in general practice (Murphy and Mattson, 1992).

The qualitative approach requires researchers to listen to people and communities in an open way. The respondents themselves can select the important questions on an issue. The validity of such research does not stem from statistical generalization but on logic other than probability theory. Qualitative studies allow a better understanding of why people think and act in the way they do and allow them to express their needs freely. This approach allows people to feel actively involved rather than being passive providers of information. It can provide information on sensitive topics (Currer, 1991). It is flexible and allows the research design, the sample, the topics to be covered, and the means of exploring these topics to be amended during the research process in the light of earlier findings (Crabtree and Miller, 1992; Pope and Mays, 1995).

Qualitative research will not establish how many people in a locality need a particular kind of service, but it will provide a sense of the range of perceived health needs within the area, the relative importance individuals attach to them, and ideas about how they can be met (Ong et al., 1992). One strategy or 'toolbox' which brings together a number of qualitative methods is rapid participatory appraisal.

Rapid participatory appraisal

Rapid appraisal techniques derived from the developing world are growing in popularity. The primary aims of rapid appraisal are to gain insight into the community's own perspective on its health and social needs; to translate these findings into joint action plans; and to establish an ongoing relationship between service purchasers, providers and the community (see below). Rapid appraisal methods have been defined as "any systematic activity designed to draw inferences, conclusions, hypotheses, or assessments, including requisition of new information in a limited period of time" (Rifkin, 1992). These appraisal methods rest on two principles (Chambers, 1983):

- *Optimal ignorance*, which demands that information which is not relevant to the objectives of the collection exercise be ignored

- *Proportionate accuracy*, which demands that the accuracy of information be kept in proportion to its use and time is not 'wasted' in validating information which serves no purpose.

In the health field, two distinct approaches have emerged. The rapid collection of quantitative epidemiological data is often called 'rapid assessment' (or 'rapid epidemiological assessment'). The other approach, called rapid appraisal (or participatory rural appraisal), is rooted in the field of rural agricultural development. This approach is characterized as one which stresses information gathering as a process which is iterative, innovative, interactive, informal, and in the field.

The scientific rigour and validity of the approach depends on the concept of triangulation, with data collection from one source being validated or rejected by checking it with data from at least two other sources or methods of collection. Through cross-checking observations among divergent data sources, apparent differences may resolve themselves and a coherent interpretation may be constructed (Brody, 1992). Informants are not selected randomly, but 'purposefully' or strategically (Johnson, 1990). Thus the people who are thought to be in the best position to understand the issues are asked. Confirming and disconfirming opinions are sought.

The attitudes and skills necessary for rapid appraisal include a willingness to learn from local people, careful listening during interviews and informal conversations, awareness and sensitivity to everything that can be directly observed, and the use of common sense in analysing the information.

Data are collected from three main sources:

- Existing written records about the neighbourhood

- Interviews with a range of informants

- Observations made in the neighbourhood or in the homes of interviewees.

From the information thus collected, an information 'pyramid' can be assembled describing the neighbourhood's problems and priorities. Potential solutions for them can be drafted (Figure 4). The bottom layer defines the composition of the community, how it is organized, and its capacities to act. The second layer covers the socio-ecological factors which influence health. The next layer covers data on the existence, coverage, accessibility and acceptability of services, allows direct evaluation of present provision, and provides a method of selecting indicators for change. The final level is concerned with national, regional and local policies that tell whether the political leadership is committed to community involvement in health. The pyramid shape is a reminder that in this method success depends on building a planning process that rests on a strong community information base. In Britain, the method has been used to define health and social needs in various communities (Cresswell, 1992; Ong et al., 1992). Application of the methods in practice is described in Chapter 4.

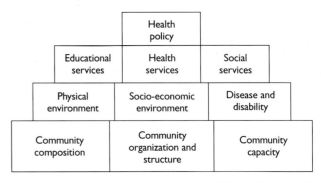

Figure 4 Information pyramid constructed for rapid appraisal

Tapping the demands, wishes and alternative perspectives of all other interested parties is sometimes called the 'corporate' approach to needs assessment (NHSME, 1991). While it may blur the differences between need and demand, or between science and vested interest, it provides other opportunities for initiating responses to the needs expressed. The key views belong to patients and elucidating them can be very difficult.

Use of survey instruments

Surveys focus on 'felt' need or individuals' own perceived needs. General practice based surveys have usually explored patients' views on the services they receive. Similar issues recur (NHS Training Division, 1994): accessibility, communication deficits, waiting times in the surgery, and satisfaction. Many recent studies have included a quality of life instrument to assess the health status of the survey population (Hunt et al., 1985).

Sykes et al. (1992) suggested that a survey is appropriate when:

- There is a recognized need for measurement of the incidence or prevalence of conditions and of the relationships between them

- Information needs are sufficiently well defined to allow the development of a structured questionnaire

- Respondents are likely to be able and willing to provide the information under the constrained circumstances of a structured survey.

The Health and Lifestyle Survey 1984 repeated in 1991 (Health Promotion Research Trust, 1993), and the General Household Survey (OPCS, 1993) yield national estimates of health status. District-based surveys have been used to compare the health of people living in small neighbourhoods with the health status of larger populations (Hume, 1995).

Recent reviews of quality of life measurement scales have found conceptual confusion reflected in many instruments (Bowling, 1991; Gill, 1994). Wilkin et al. (1992) have drawn up a guide to 40 measures of health status suitable for use in varying degrees in primary care research and practice. They include sections dealing with physical function, mental health and social support. Multidimensional and disease-specific measures are available. Need is defined as a measurable deficiency from a goal and every measure implies value judgements about what are appropriate goals and what constitutes deficiency from the goal.

The Nottingham Health Profile is a well established British multidimensional measure of perceived health (Hunt et al., 1986). It has 38 items and is easy to complete. Scores on six dimensions of health are produced: energy, emotional reaction, social isolation, sleep, pain and physical mobility. Hopton et al. (1991), in a study of the working patterns of 85 general practitioners, found that significant differences were found according to age, sex and illness status, length of consultation, and doctors' perception of the presence of psychosocial illness. The high number of zero scorers resulted in a skewed distribution, and the instrument has proved rather insensitive to small degrees of perceived ill health. It suffers from a number of weaknesses. It is not a measure of health but a measure of distress; its content is more relevant to people suffering from chronic illnesses than to general populations. Analysis and interpretation can be difficult.

The Short Form 36 health survey questionnaire (SF 36) is able to detect low levels of ill health in patients who score 0 (good health) on the Nottingham Health Profile (Brazier et al., 1992). The SF 36 has been applied in general practice. In a survey of 1700 patients in the north east of Scotland, the SF 36 was again found to be acceptable to patients, internally consistent, and valid as a measure of the health status of a wide range of patients (Garratt et al., 1993). The SF 36 can be used with a condition-specific measure of clinical outcome to monitor a specific patient group. Health status instruments may be used in population surveys as well as in individual patient care (Fitzpatrick et al., 1992).

Walsh (1994) studied data from a large postal survey about back pain using general practice age-sex registers as the sampling frame, and inspected the general practice records of sub-samples of respondents and non-respondents. Such registers can provide a suitable sampling frame for epidemiological purposes and general practice records can be useful in assessing response bias in health surveys. The use of general practice lists is likely to present more difficulties where many practices serve an area or where a high proportion of the population is not registered with a general practitioner. Surveys of patients' perceptions of need for primary health care services suggest that priority rankings may differ between the healthy and unhealthy subgroups (Hopton and Dlugolecka, 1995). To promote equity some opinions may have to be given greater weight.

Higher response rates may result from letters sent by the general practitioner than to letters from local research institutions (Smith, 1985). The response rate can also be improved by sending reminders, by enclosing prepaid envelopes, and by financial inducements, but it seems little affected by the length of the questionnaire, the use of pre-coded responses or a personalized accompanying letter (Cartwright, 1986). Low response rates are commoner among men, individuals of lower social class, poor education and younger age (Sheikh and Mattingly, 1981).

It is essential to pilot any questionnaire that has not been used before. Where response rates are low, it may be worth sampling the records of non-responders to explore the ways in which your responders are unrepresentative. Table 6 lists areas which may be profitably explored using a practice-based postal survey.

Table 6 Possible postal survey topics

- Chronic illness
  —any long-term illness
  —several marker conditions, e.g. hypertension, back pain
- Acute illnesses and experience of common symptoms
- Consider a general health status instrument, e.g. SF36, NHP
- Consider a disease-specific instrument
- Use of health services over the last 6 or 12 months
- Perceived need for current and potential services
- Social and demographic characteristics
  —car or house ownership, unemployment
- Specific concerns and worries which may affect health
- Specific questions for people with specific long-term health problems or carers
- Patient satisfaction

Patient participation

The Royal College of General Practitioners (RCGP) has long encouraged patient participation in general practice (Pritchard, 1981; Heritage, 1994). In 1983, the RCGP set up the Patients' Liaison Group, consisting of seven general practitioners and seven lay people. Its remit was "to feed back to Council areas of patient concern". The College has published a third edition of its 'start up' guide for those interested in forming a patient participation group (Pritchard, 1993).

Community participation is a process in which local people are actively involved in discussion and activities to identify their needs and bring about improvements in the health of the community (Oakley, 1989). The NHS Management Executive (1992) has detailed how purchasers can involve the community in deciding service priorities in various ways. *Local Voices* contains many examples from the field of primary care. However, the concept of community participation is poorly understood by most people working in primary care (Gooding, 1991). Health professionals have not been trained to promote community involvement, although free-standing community health projects have successfully involved the public in assessing need (Kennedy, 1994). Work with a variety of groups representing different community interest is frequently challenging and demands managerial skills of a high order. Health professionals may need to relinquish established attitudes and behaviours in order to meet the challenge of encouraging local people to help in the organizational setting. Doctors need to be confident in the management of their practice. Without this confidence, it is hard to invite potentially critical feedback from patients. On the other hand, without community participation, needs assessment remains a purely professional exercise generating only normative priorities in Bradshaw's terms.

Summary

Different approaches to the assessment of need have been described. These are complementary and in practice a combination of approaches is required. The data available to support practice-based needs assessment can be overwhelming. Some is of doubtful relevance. There are clearly dangers in relying on subjective assessments. The key to successful health needs analysis therefore lies in reconciling different sources of information—'triangulation'. A comprehensive assessment brings together both qualitative and quantitative data. The use of different data in practice is illustrated in Chapter 4.

Needs assessment in practice

I N THIS chapter, case studies are used to illustrate the approaches described above. They do not claim to provide models or 'gold standards' but to demonstrate achievements and issues faced in practice. These examples demonstrate a significant degree of overlap with many teams using a combination of approaches.

PRACTICE-BASED APPROACHES

Health needs assessment: the team approach
(Schofield, 1992)

Aim

To create a profile of a community and its health needs by a primary health care team using data from the different disciplines represented in the team.

Background

Schofield has contrasted the rhetoric of collaboration and teamwork in general practice with the reality of fragmented community services, medical domination of the agenda, and services provided in inverse proportion to need. However, he has provided an example of the way a team began to assess the needs of the practice population and set its own priorities. Each discipline contributed its own distinctive perspective on which patients can benefit from care.

Methods

Table 7 shows the range of topics and the sources of information brought together by the primary health care team to create a profile of the community. No one discipline could do this alone, although the experience of health visitors creating community profiles was a particularly valuable resource in this exercise.

Table 7 Range of topics and sources of information utilized by Schofield (1992) to construct a practice profile

Topic	Sources of information
A. Population	
Population	Practice register
Population characteristics	Census
Housing	Local authorities
Transport	Local authorities
Facilities	Health visitor profile
Future developments	County plan
B. Health status	
Causes of death	Practice register
Child health	Child health computer, health visitor records
Teenage health	School practice register
Family planning	Practice register, DHA clinics
Maternity	Midwife, health visitor records
Adult screening	Practice register
Chronic diseases	Practice register
Mental health	Practice register, community mental health
Mental handicap	Mental handicap team
Chronic disabilities	Social services
Hospital admissions	Practice register, waiting list
Elderly	Elderly surveillance, home care services

Results

Table 8 shows some of the problem areas or needs that this exercise identified.

Table 8 Problems identified

1. High proportion of elderly people in the population
2. Lack of housing affordable by young families
3. No direct bus to local district hospital
4. A high proportion of elderly patients dying in hospital (including a community hospital) (63%)
5. A low rate of mothers starting to breast feed (59%)
6. A low uptake of family planning services (25%) and a high rate of terminations of pregnancy in teenagers (15 per 1000)
7. A high rate of overdoses (2 per 1000) particularly in the 16–24 age group

Lessons learnt

- Needs assessment can be performed by doctors, but a primary health care team brings a wider vision to assess the needs of the population and to respond flexibly to meet those needs.

- Small numbers diminish the confidence that can be placed in some items and make comparisons with district-based data and comparisons from year to year unreliable. However, even a single death from cervical cancer in a woman who had never been screened concentrates the whole team on the importance of achieving these targets.

- Some of the problems that affect the population, for example housing and transport, are not the direct responsibility of the primary health care team but have a major impact on the way in which it plans and delivers services. There is therefore a role for the team to act as an advocate to other organizations.

- Other problems such as family planning or termination of pregnancy were initially seen entirely as health service issues. However, their identification led to the formation of a multidisciplinary group. As well as health professionals, this included teachers, youth workers, social workers and parents, who took a much broader view of the problems of teenage pregnancy and its possible solutions.

Case-finding and proactive care
(Hart et al., 1991)

Aim

To improve the health in a practice's registered population by identifying treatable problems and risk factors at an early stage, to audit the findings, and to enter into repeated cycles of case finding and audit.

Background

Hart's paper described an attempt, sustained over 25 years, to provide whole population care as well as general medical services to 1800 people registered in a small Welsh village.

Methods

Between 1968 and 1970, 98% of the population aged 20 to 64 years were screened for high blood pressure, mainly by case-finding within consultations but supplemented by active call-up and finally by home visits.

Similar but less energetic approaches were later applied to older patients, and to other coronary risk factors: cigarette smoking, serum total cholesterol concentration, obesity, diabetes, airways obstruction, and alcohol problems.

Major tasks included the employment and training of practice staff, the conversion to A4 records and computerization.

Results

The proportion of men aged 20 to 64 years who said they smoked fell from 61% (290/476) in 1968–70 to 36% (162/456) in 1985, whereas the proportion of women who smoked was unchanged: 43% (187/436) in 1968–70 and 42% (190/448) in 1985. In 116 screened hypertensive patients, group mean blood pressure fell from 186/110 mm Hg before treatment to 146/84 mm Hg, as did the proportion of smokers (56% v 20%), but body mass index and total cholesterol concentration showed no significant change. In 34 diabetic patients mean blood pressure and the proportion of smokers fell (171/93 mm Hg v 155/81 mm Hg; 44% v 12%). The age standardized mortality ratio in 1981–86 was lower than in a neighbouring village without a developed case-finding programme (actual to expected deaths <65 = 21 to 22 in Glyncorrwg, 48 to 30 in control village).

Lessons learnt

- Whole population care through organized case-finding and audit is feasible but only with a labour-intensive, structured approach combining accessibility, flexibility and continuity of care.

- Despite shortcomings, the available data were consistent with the hypothesis that whole population care helps reduce mortality. Achieving a reduction in smoking in the general population was more difficult than in the target groups of hypertensive and diabetic patients.

- Continuing care is more difficult and demanding than case finding. Clinics are important for chronic disease management. Protected time, delegation to nurses and specialized training for them, recognition of defaulters and shared learning in groups of patients with common problems are essential to controlling chronic conditions. They required the organization of clinics for hypertensive and diabetic patients. Other cardiovascular risks, airways obstruction, epilepsy and alcohol problems were handled more effectively by extending consultation time and referral to the practice nurse.

- The work involved in meeting the sum of many individuals' health needs in this way is enormous and has to be resourced. The much criticized banding scheme was an attempt to provide incentives for this work. Recent studies have highlighted the limits to practice-based risk factor intervention. Such work cannot be assumed to be cost-effective (Fowler and Mant, 1990).

Meeting health care needs in a deprived community
(Marsh and Channing, 1988)

Aim

This paper is cited as an example of a primary health care team responding effectively to health needs identified through systematic study of their records. The ability to respond to identified need must be borne in mind when selecting the methods by which to assess need. The aim of the initiative was to narrow the 'health gap' between deprived and endowed communities in the practice catchment area.

Background

There is considerable evidence that clinic-based and opportunistic screening programmes fail to reach those most at risk. This practice was concerned about the low uptake of preventive services among the most deprived members of the practice population and devised a successful strategy for tackling the problems.

Methods

First a systematic study was made of the practice records, comparing groups of 'deprived' patients from a local authority housing estate within the area with an 'endowed' group matched for age and sex living in a pleasant private housing estate in another part of the practice.

It was subsequently decided that the existing system of "informal extra effort—health visitors spending more time in the area, paying opportunistic attention to the deprived families when they presented, and the presence of a small peripheral community clinic operated by the district health authority" was failing to provide adequate preventive care for the deprived community.

Results

It was found that the practice's deprived patients had:

- More serious physical illness

- More hospital admissions

- More casualty attendances

- More mental illness

- More referrals to consultants

- More general practice consultations

- Fewer childhood immunizations

- More teenage pregnancies

- More pregnancies terminated

- Fewer cervical smears among the older women

- Lower attendance for preventive health checks

- More smokers.

An intensive programme was therefore adopted aimed at the deprived group, which including the following elements:

- A prevention card covering smoking status, tetanus immunization, blood pressure measurement, urine tests, attendance at well-man and well-women clinics, family planning advice, cervical smear tests, and childhood immunizations was attached to the front of the records of each patient in the deprived community.

- The card prompted doctors to discuss any outstanding preventive care at each consultation.

- Copies of the updated cards were supplied to the health visitors for use on home visits.

- Letters were sent to the senior female member of each household describing the practice policy on preventive care and listing the preventive record for each member of the household.

- Progress was monitored every three months, and each doctor was issued with a set of tables showing coverage of the various items of preventive care.

- Progress and problems were discussed regularly at practice meetings.

- Pre-arranged home visits were made jointly by doctors and health visitors to provide preventive care to those who failed to attend the relevant clinics.

Lessons learnt

As a result of this focused programme it was possible to improve the following:

- Childhood immunization coverage

- Cervical smear rates

- Anti-tetanus immunization coverage

- Blood pressure measurement

- Urine analysis

- Attendance at preventive health checks

- Recording of smoking habits.

By the end of the 15-month programme, the deprived patients had a better record for many of the preventive procedures than the endowed group.

COMPARATIVE APPROACHES

General practice morbidity networks

Aim

To improve the collection and transfer of high quality data in primary care by developing/coding standard datasets for use in assessing health needs, audit and service planning.

Background

Although systems have been developed to assist clinical management within practices, sharing of comparative data is difficult given the diversity of different systems in use. In 1988, the Joint Computing Group of the RCGP and the GMSC recommended the Read codes for the standard classification of general practice data. This allows access to a thesaurus of medical terms expressed in language suitable for general practitioners based on a hierarchical structure (Chisholm, 1990). The intention with Read coding was to produce comprehensive information about individual patients allowing clinical physicians to be better informed and, by ensuring compatibility, to allow comparison of data for assessment and audit of health needs (NHS Centre for Coding and Classification, 1993). Accurate and comprehensive data would also provide the sampling framework for clinical and organizational research and development. The Department of Health subsequently purchased the Read clinical coding classification and the National Coding Centre at Loughborough was established to maintain and develop the codes.

Several networks have now been established in different parts of the country to optimize the use of data collected routinely in general practice. Three well-known initiatives are discussed below.

Methods

1. LAPIS (SHEFFIELD)

The Sheffield Health Information Project (SHIP) has gained considerable experience linking many data sources to individuals on its population health register (Payne et al., 1994a). As a pilot site for the District Information Systems Project, Sheffield has a rich source of health event data, most of which includes an identifier for the patient's general practice.

An ideal practice population health information system should have the following attributes:

- The information should refer to practices' populations of registered patients.

- The information system should be easy to use.

- Comparisons between one practice and other practices should be possible.

- Other comparisons, for example, admission rates related to proportion of elderly patients, should be possible.

Working closely with the family health services authority (FHSA), and particularly using the FHSA population register, a locality and practice information system (LAPIS) has been constructed which brings together a wide variety of health information (Table 9). The system is developed in the Excel Macro language, providing a standalone application which the user runs by pointing and clicking on a series of menu screens. For any data item, the user is offered a choice of a ranked bar graph, together with a tabulation of the data itself. The system also allows clusters of practices to be identified and compared, for example on a geographical basis.

Figure 5 shows the crude all-cause mortality rate in Sheffield practices based on the period 1987 to 1991. The

Table 9 Data sources available

Practice population structure (obtained from FHSA register)
Total population size
Proportion aged 0–64, 65–74, 75+

Hospital health event data
(obtained from district information system)
All-cause admission rate
Admission rate for asthma, coronary heart disease, stroke,
    mental health problems, respiratory disease, and so on
A&E attendance rate
Outpatient attendance rate by specialty

Community health service data
District nursing service contracts

Items of service data
(obtained from the FHSA returns)
Night-visit rates
Vaccination and immunization rates

Prescribing data (from PACT)

Health visitor data (obtained from health visitor returns for
families with children 0–5)
Breast feeding
Proportion on income support
Ethnic minority proportion

Mortality data (from FHSA register linked with OPCS death
returns)
All-cause mortality
Cause-specific mortality—for example, coronary heart disease,
    stroke, respiratory disease, and so on

Attributed data (information available only on a locality basis
but attributed to each practice in relation to the proportion of
patients registered living in that electoral ward)
Unemployment rate
Long-standing chronic illness
Ethnicity
Jarman and Townsend scores

practice of interest is highlighted (practice X) together
with Sheffield and sector means. This particular practice
has a substantially higher mortality rate than many.

Figure 6 shows a scatterplot of one variable versus
another, which indicates that this particular practice also
has a high proportion of its population aged over 75
years. In the graph each Sheffield practice can be compared both in respect of mortality rate and its proportion
of patients over 75.

When released to individual practices and non-district
health authority agencies in the city, the practices are
anonymized using numerical codes. The practice is told
only its own identifying code and is thus able to compare
itself with others without breaking confidentiality.
Practices are, of course, free to tell each other their identifying codes and have usually been keen to do this. The
latest version is distributed with a 'toolkit' setting out
principles and practical advice about needs assessment.

Practices have been keen to exploit the added insight
which the system can give to their work. Releasing such
information might be seen by some as liable to cause problems. However, experience indicates that general practitioners will respond to an open approach and to a system
which is already designed to allow them access.

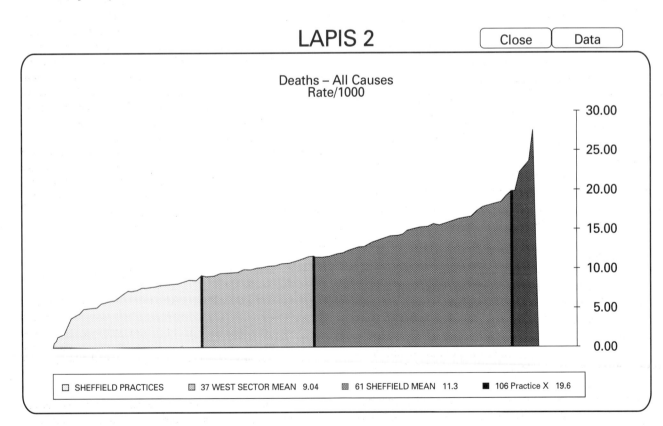

Figure 5 All-cause mortality rate

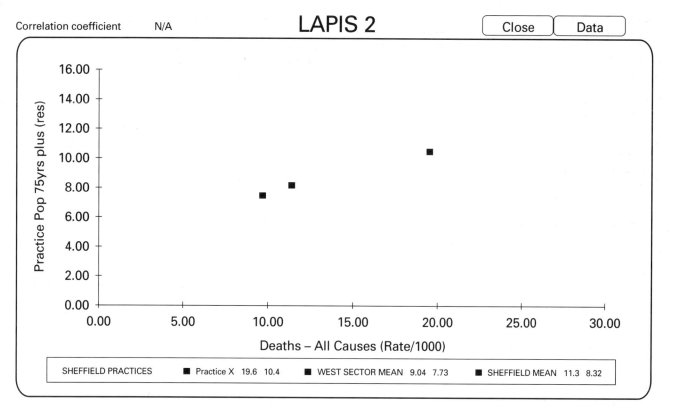

Figure 6   Scatterplot of age versus mortality

2. WAPPCHIP

The Wakefield and Pontefract Primary Care Health Information Project was formed in April 1992 (Smith et al., 1995). It consisted of a network of 10 practices and representatives from public health medicine, the FHSA and researchers from the University of Leeds. A working group developed a standard dataset to provide a consistent and uniform approach to data collection. The items in the dataset were defined by reference to practice demography, morbidity and lifestyles which the working group agreed were of value to practices for planning purposes.

Matching the dataset with the Read codes raised several problems including the lack of a hierarchical structure, the absence of adequate coding for family history of certain morbidity, the lack of standard definitions for data about lifestyle, inconsistencies in codes for recording the outcomes, and difficulties in coding for severity of some morbidities.

One of the aims of WAPPCHIP was to develop new methodologies for health needs assessment. For example, WAPPCHIP practices provided data from consultations to ascertain the prevalence of musculoskeletal conditions and associated disability. The project results were used for comparison with other published evidence of prevalence and disability to determine general practitioner management, referral patterns, and service deficiencies in the Wakefield area, in order to inform planning. The study formed the basis for the development of a community-based rheumatology service including the appointment of a community-based consultant rheumatologist (Wilson, 1995).

3. MIQUEST

This project was funded by the NHSE Information Management Group. A structured Health Query Language (HQL) was defined. The HQL is capable of expressing many current and potential requirements for data extraction from the following general practice computer systems: EMIS, AAH Meditel and Genisyst. Windows software was developed for creating and editing HQL queries, as well as managing the distribution of queries and the aggregation of responses. Individual or aggregated responses can be incorporated into widely available databases, spreadsheets and statistical packages. MIQUEST is being used in several health authorities and practices in England and Wales for health needs assessment (see page 43 for details). The MEDICS scheme in Northumberland and the Lancashire Morbidity Data Collection Project provide examples.

Lessons learnt

- Information networks such as LAPIS can provide both health authorities and general practitioners with a wealth of information without involving the practices themselves in any extra work. They may encourage a population approach to health at primary care level. They will serve both as a stimulus and a vehicle for the collection and presentation of new primary care data.

- These projects have raised awareness amongst participating practices about the importance of collecting accurate and reliable data. Many practices have begun to recognize the value of agreed clinical definitions and are developing practice guidelines to ensure consistency within the team.

- Use of the computer has many advantages in the recording and analysis of health promotion information especially if data entry is standardized. Opportunistic health prompts will allow the targeting of relevant health promotion activity to the individual, at-risk patient when he/she attends the surgery. However, practices will need to devise alternative health promotion initiatives for people who do not attend, otherwise there is a risk that some patients, particularly male, may be disadvantaged.

- Difficulties with the coding system must be addressed if the potential of information from primary care is to be realized. The use of qualifiers may create more flexible ways of representing clinical terms (DoH, 1993b) but systems must be user friendly. Some of these problems may be addressed in the latest version of the Read codes.

- Comparative data often provide the first pointers for further audit/needs analysis.

- Participation in a morbidity network can be the prelude to more extensive joint working. Most of the WAPPCHIP practices are now part of a local fund-holding consortium.

- The experience accruing from many data collection schemes round the country needs to be shared more systematically. Central investment may be required to co-ordinate this.

Performance indicators for general practice
(Old et al., 1994)

Aim

To develop and pilot the use of practice activity indicators to assist in practice audit and planning.

Background

Some health authorities are now producing performance indicators for the practices they administer (Hanlon and Hargreaves, 1994; Payne et al., 1994a; Majeed and Voss, 1995). The Inter-Authority Comparisons and Consultancy, Health Services Management Centre (University of Birmingham) in conjunction with the Southampton Health Commission has developed a standalone PC-based indicator package using routine data sources (Old et al., 1994). Table 10 lists the areas covered. This can provide a more detailed picture of a practice's performance allowing debate about its strengths and weaknesses.

Table 10   Indicator subject areas

• Patient-based indicators	• Staff ratios
• Cytology	• Immunization and
• Prescribing	vaccination rates
• Minor surgery	• Night visits
• Outpatient referrals	• Inpatient admissions
• Maternity and family planning	

Many general practitioners view the development of such management tools as threatening. They raise the spectre of league tables of practice performance and must be used and interpreted appropriately. General practitioners need to collaborate with health boards and health authorities to refine such packages and improve their usefulness.

Results

No formal evaluation of the impact of such indicators has yet been undertaken. However, experience with PACT data suggests that doctors will respond to comparison with their own practice's activities by effecting change. The response from practices in health commissions using this package has so far been positive. Such routine data can beg new questions but may assist directly in planning decisions.

Two examples are given below.

1. NIGHT VISITS

One particular practice had been concerned about the high number of night visits it was undertaking. However, analysis showed that while it had a slightly above average number of visits per general practitioner, the visits per head of population were close to the average. The practice population was thus not unduly demanding, but the fact that the general practitioners within the practice were doing all their own night visits may have partly explained their sense of being overworked.

2. CERVICAL CYTOLOGY

Another practice appeared to be having great success in achieving its targets for cytology and immunization. The practice had recently achieved uptakes of 100% on immunization and 90% on cytology. However, the practice also had the highest proportion of inadequate smears of any practice in the area. The practice comprised a single-handed female general practitioner with a high level of nursing support. The practice nurse was assisting with the smears but needed further training.

Lessons learnt

- Comparative indices of need such as this will require careful interpretation. They measure only certain aspects of performance. For example, a simple referral rate says nothing about the appropriateness of these referrals. Performance indicators generally say little about primary health care teams' most important role: the clinical care of individual patients.

- Performance indicators in their present state of development should be used only for audit and planning within the practice. Rewarding 'high performing practices' with increased allocations for staff or premises would create a perverse incentive by attracting attention from the quality of clinical care.

- Performance indicators are constructed from routine data in which there may be errors (for example, inflation of list sizes, under-enumeration of census data, inaccurate coding). Health authorities will need to be aware of these limitations if using such indicators to monitor general practice. General practitioners must be involved at all stages in their development and implementation (Majeed and Voss, 1995).

- General practitioners can benefit from performance indicators. They can use them to identify how their practice deviates from the norm and where scope for further investigation and audit may exist. Performance indicators can also help practices to identify priorities for improvement and to monitor how well they address them over time. Finally, performance indicators can be used to carry out descriptive research into variations in medical practice in primary care (Baker and Klein, 1991).

PUBLIC HEALTH APPROACHES

Use of 'indicative prevalences' for assessing morbidity and health promotion needs
(Charlton et al., 1994)

Aims

To construct indicative prevalences for a range of diseases and risk markers and use them in planning health promotion interventions.

Background

Health promotion has become an increasingly important part of primary health care. However, with limited time, resources or evidence for the effectiveness of many preventive interventions, it is important to set priorities.

The 1990 General Practitioner Contract incorporated many preventive elements: child health surveillance, annual screening for patients over 75-years-old, target payments for immunization of cervical cytology, and health promotion clinics. The quality and uptake of clinics was uneven and unrelated to the health needs of practice populations (Gillam, 1992b). The banding scheme and chronic disease management payments were introduced in 1993 (NHSME, 1993b).

Charlton et al. (1994) have shown how practice data can be used to set priorities by generating 'indicative prevalences' for a hypothetical average general practice, with a list size of 10 000 in Newcastle upon Tyne. Indicative prevalences are measures of point prevalence, incidence and mortality rates generated for disease, and risk markers. Conditions reflected key areas in the *Health of the Nation* document (DoH, 1992).

Indicative prevalences can similarly be used to compare data submitted by practices under the banding and chronic disease management schemes.

Methods

Data for indicative prevalences were derived from three main sources:

- Newcastle Health and Lifestyle Survey 1991

- OPCS death rates for 1988-1992

- Regional health authority hospital admissions data.

Census data for 1991 were used to calculate incidence and prevalences. The age structure of the hypothetical population reflected that of Newcastle as a whole. Direct standardization was used in most cases to provide the indicative prevalences.

Age-specific rates for men and women in 10-year bands were applied to the hypothetical practice to give the expected number of people with the condition or factor in their practice population. These numbers were summed to give an overall practice figure.

Results

Table 11 lists some of the indicative prevalences described. They varied widely and were highest for risk markers such as failure to exercise adequately, moderate to extreme obesity and smoking. Common diseases such as angina and diabetes are of intermediate prevalence. Some *Health of the Nation* priorities are rare (deaths from cervical cancer, malignant melanoma or suicide). They constitute a relatively small burden compared with the mass of hidden markers that may lead to disease.

Table 11 Indicative prevalences

Condition	Scale of problem
*Smoking:**	
Never smoked	2830 people at any one time
Former smoker	1969 people at any one time
Smoker	1512 people at any one time
Cardiovascular disease:	
Angina	175 people at any one time
Family history of premature myocardial infarction*	1715 people at any one time
Myocardial infarction deaths	18 deaths/year
Myocardial infarction survivors*	347 people at any one time
Coronary artery bypass grafts	3 operations/year
Hypertension	1145 people at any one time
Transient ischaemic attack incidence	4 new cases/year
Stroke incidence	20 people/year
Stroke deaths	18 deaths/year
Exercise target:[*†]	
Achieved	617 people at any one time
Not achieved	6871 people at any one time
*Body mass index (weight (kg)/height (m)^2):**[✦]	
Normal	4703 people at any one time
Moderate obesity	2183 people at any one time
Extreme obesity	602 people at any one time
Alcohol consumption:[*††]	
Safe	5920 people at any one time
Hazardous	1285 people at any one time
Dangerous	283 people at any one time
Diabetes mellitus:	
Prevalence*	165 people at any one time
Deaths	1 death/year
Asthma:	
Admissions	41 people/year
Deaths	3 deaths/10 years

*Only people aged 16–74 years.

† >12 occasions of vigorous activity in past 4 weeks for 16–54 year olds

✦ Normal < 25, moderate obesity 25–39, extreme obesity >39

†† Safe < 22 units/week (< 15 for women), hazardous 22–50 (15–35 for women); dangerous < 50 (< 35 for women).

Lessons learnt

- Primary health care teams can use indicative prevalences to examine national priorities in the light of their own patients' probable needs. The same methods can be applied to generate practice-specific information on expected prevalence, incidence and mortality.

- The systematic identification and management of patients with hypertension, angina and previous myocardial infarction are high priorities for secondary prevention in primary care. The benefits of prophylactic aspirin and/or beta blockers in preventing the recurrence of myocardial infarction are well established.

- Health promotion activities should be planned on the basis of prevalence of risk factors and conditions. These are limited by the lack of information on the cost-effectiveness of interventions. The OXCHECK and Family Heart Studies provided some evidence of the effectiveness of practice nurses in effecting improvements in diastolic blood pressure, serum cholesterol and weight gain (Wood et al., 1994; ICRF, 1995). Their impact on smoking behaviour was disappointing. However, there is evidence that brief interventions from general practitioners can reduce both smoking and hazardous alcohol consumption (NHSE, 1995).

- A focus on personal interventions in general practice is likely to be more effective and cheaper than universal screening and advice. An organized team with efficient information systems is necessary to achieve high coverage.

Community-oriented primary care
(Gillam et al., 1994)

Aim

To improve the practice population's health through targeted interventions selected on the basis of systematic needs assessment.

Background

Community-oriented primary care (COPC) has been defined as the provision of primary care services to a defined community, coupled with systematic efforts to identify and address the major health problems of that community through effective modifications to services provided (Nutting, 1987). COPC was developed by Kark and others in rural South Africa (Kark, 1981), Israel (Abramson, 1988) and the USA (Wright, 1993). The basic concepts are familiar (White, 1976; Geiger, 1983) and have been practised for many years by family practitioners in the UK. Tudor Hart's studies of heart disease prevention are examples of community-oriented family practice (Hart, 1990a).

The King's Fund has developed COPC for use in the UK as a possible vehicle for developing primary care-led commissioning. The importance of public health skills in general practice is increasingly recognized (Handysides, 1994) and COPC may offer an appropriate methodology for helping develop them. The King's Fund COPC 'package' includes educational materials for use in structured workshops with practice-based teams and DHA/FHSA managers and a programme for COPC developers from local agencies planning to introduce, support, and extend COPC in their areas.

Methods

The King's Fund COPC programme began in four pilot sites (Haringey, Northumberland, Sheffield, and Winchester), when workshops were organized for two or three local practices and DHA/FHSA staff. Primary health care teams worked through the stages of the COPC cycle (Figure 7) in order to provide an understanding of the approach, build commitment, and enable participants to relay their experience to the rest of their team.

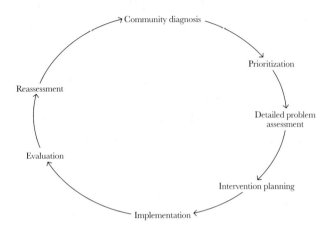

Figure 7   The COPC cycle

THE COPC CYCLE

An assessment of the practice population's health needs is carried out in three stages.

First, the primary health care team defines the health problems of its community on the basis of available quantitative and qualitative data (Table 12). This includes team members' local knowledge derived from working in the community over years. Each team produces a comprehensive list of the major health-related problems in its practice population.

Table 12   Data used for community diagnosis

1. **Practice environment:**
   e.g. physical location, topographical features, transport, physical description of surgery premises, local employment, housing, local environment risk factors

2. **Community characteristics:**
   e.g. practice list age-sex breakdown, socio-economic status, educational status, ethnic minorities (numbers and special needs), deprivation indices, unemployment rates

3. **State of health:**
   Morbidity   e.g. data on patients with chronic diseases (e.g. hypertension, heart failure, stroke, asthma, diabetes), antenatal and births data, teenage conception rates, termination rates, infectious disease notifications, specialist referral rates, inpatient admission rates
   Mortality   e.g. local ward-level standardized mortality ratios specific (e.g. coronary heart disease, lung cancer)

4. **Risk factors:**
   e.g. behavioural data on smoking, alcohol consumption, dietary, exercise patterns, substance misuse, sexual behaviour

5. **Health service system:**
   Within the practice, e.g. number of general practitioners, nurses, other practice-attached staff, special interests, complementary therapy, patient turnover rate

Outside the practice, e.g. health services (hospital and community), voluntary services (e.g. meals on wheels)—gap analysis

A great deal of data on this list will tend to be available at ward not practice level. Care is required in its interpretation.

Secondly comes prioritization. A simple grid is used to score each health problem in relation to specific criteria, namely size of problem, availability of an effective intervention, acceptability to the team and consumer, feasibility, community involvement and resource requirements (Figure 8). Primary health care teams can override the scoring system in certain instances, for example when the top priority problem is already being addressed.

- A rural practice initially ranked cardiovascular disease as its highest priority. However, members of the team felt that they were already investing a great deal of effort in this area. In discussing other priorities a practice nurse drew attention to a major cause of distress to affected patients: urinary incontinence. At first the doctors did not appreciate the extent of the problem. In the words of the nurse: "You don't see it. We're always replacing the leaflets on incontinence. They come to us". The team members elected to accept this as their priority. A prevalence study has been performed on women aged 40-49 years with a 75% response rate. The results show that only 31% have never had an episode of incontinence and that 23% could be defined as having marked incontinence. The planned intervention will include both preventive exercises, community education and the setting up of a local continence clinic by a specially trained practice nurse.

- Two inner city practices with very high rates of unemployment concluded that highest priority should be given to adolescent health. The high prevalence of cigarette smoking, drug and alcohol abuse in this age group were well established. In addition, adolescents were often caught up in the violence and social unrest afflicting the community. The extent of teenage pregnancies was realized only during the workshop.

Having selected one health problem (Table 13), the teams next explore the extent of the priority problem in the total practice population—the detailed assessment. This constitutes a baseline for later evaluation. The inclusion of non-users is a cardinal feature of COPC. The teams use their own and local expert knowledge as well as specialist literature.

Intervention plans should define relevant activities, who is responsible for their implementation, records required, training needs, milestones and deadlines. Realistic objectives must be clearly defined. District health authorities and family health services authorities have provided limited extra resources and advice for survey design, questionnaire development, data processing and analysis.

The teams then consider the methods they will use to assess the degree to which programme objectives have been met. Early definition of the data required for the evaluation is a critical part of the COPC process.

CRITERION	PROJECT					
	Coughs and colds	Postnatal depression	Carers	Asthma	Smoking	Cancer
Prevalence/incidence	3	3	3	3	3	3
Severity of problem	1	3	3	3	3	3
Effective intervention	1	3	3	3	2	1
Acceptability/feasibility	1	3	2	2	3	2
Community involvement	1	2	3	2	2	2
Costs and resources	3	2	2	2	2	2
TOTAL SCORE	10	16	16	15	15	13

Figure 8 Sample prioritization grid

Table 13 Community-oriented primary care project topics

Smoking
Cardiovascular risk factors in middle age
Urinary incontinence
Health behaviours in adolescence
Depression in women
School health
People taking minor tranquillizers
Hypertension in ethnic minorities

In the final reassessment phase a decision is made as to whether or not to continue the particular intervention in the light of the evaluation. The community diagnosis is revisited prior to re-entering the COPC cycle.

- A fundholding urban practice has used the COPC process imaginatively. Beginning with a single project on hypertension, the team has moved on to identify a range of subjects for investigation and intervention. This now includes asthmatics, elderly people with special needs, mothers with young babies and the bereaved. The presentation of an individual clinical case problem at a practice meeting elicits the question: what is the extent of the problem in the community as a whole? All staff are involved in the decision-making process.

Results

Participation in the COPC project has helped develop skills in protocol development, needs assessment, project management, monitoring, and evaluation. The case studies illustrate the potential role of the COPC process in defining hitherto 'neglected' health problems in a community. However, this work is time-consuming. Assessment of health needs at practice level requires the collation of many and various sources of data. The intimate knowledge of a neighbourhood derived from years at the coalface is easily undervalued. Often, it cannot be bettered. The contribution of community nursing staff is particularly important. Generally, COPC appeared to increase mutual understanding among participants of each other's roles. The state of development of practice information systems is an important factor affecting the momentum of the project. The discipline of focused data collection, analysis and evaluation developed computer literacy among key individuals.

Health of the Nation priorities may not apply equally in all practice populations. Ownership is critical to the success of innovative preventive work in general practice. Many general practitioners feel 'over-managed'. The sense of greater autonomy that COPC can provide is in itself motivating for primary health care teams.

The COPC cycle is closely akin to a conventional management or audit cycle. What distinguishes it from most practice-based audit is its starting point. Traditionally, in selecting audit topics, doctors have begun with concerns of their own. COPC uses a more objective community profiling exercise against which to select priorities.

The pilot project has demonstrated that COPC can offer a useful framework for fundholding practices seeking to develop needs-led purchasing plans. The principles underlying it may also be relevant to the development of locality purchasing where systematic approaches to the assessment of small areas' health needs are often lacking.

Finally, the practice projects yielded quantifiable benefits for patients. Interventions yielding small health gains at practice level (for example, 31 smokers quitting) may nonetheless be extremely cost-effective.

Lessons learnt

- A commitment to improve the whole practice population's health requires an understanding of those not in regular contact with the practice. COPC enables primary health care teams to adopt a systematic approach to community health needs assessment, prioritization of local health problems, and the identification of effective health interventions based on sound research.

- Primary health care teams that can apply public health frameworks to their work will better understand the commissioning process.

Mapping health care needs of the practice population
(Colledge and Morse, 1995)

Aims

1. To develop a practice profile by modelling the primary health care database using a geographic information system (GIS) mapping software, combined with census and epidemiological data.

2. To develop a qualitative data pack to be used by health visitors and other members of the primary health care team for evaluation of patient satisfaction and health care needs on a continuing basis.

Background

Ballantrae lies in the far south of Ayrshire. The socio-economic status of the population is evenly distributed. Housing stock is good, the environment is pleasant and the weather relatively mild (for Scotland). The population of Ballantrae and the surrounding district is about 1500.

The geographical study of disease and health has a long history when dealing with the tracing of epidemics but the application of GIS to facilitate health needs assessment is a relatively new development. Recently disease-mapping, especially of mortality and morbidity with special reference to cancer research, has been developed (Boyle et al., 1989).

Methods

A Geographic Information System (GIS) is an integrated package of geographical mapping utilities and a database of spatially referenced attributes. Since a good deal of the data used and generated by a general practice and its patients have a spatial dimension, a GIS may be particularly useful to primary health care teams.

There is a variety of GIS packages available, designed to handle varying amounts and types of data simultaneously. MapInfo was used here. It can be run on a portable or desktop personal computer and offers:

- Quick and easy access to large volumes of data with the ability to
  —select detail by area or theme
  —link or merge datasets
  —analyse spatial characteristics of data

—search for particular characteristics or features in an area

—update data quickly and cheaply

—model data and assess alternatives

- Flexible forms of output, including:
  —maps
  —graphs
  —address lists.

Results

From the database in the practice, a pilot map of the practice population by post code units was developed. This identified the territorial boundaries of the practice.

Into these post code units a map was created of the 1991 census population and then a thematic map of the actual patient population (Figure 9). From this exercise it was then possible to search any local settlement served by the practice and establish the population as at the 1991 census against the actual number of patients registered by the practice. From the census data, the range of the total population in the practice catchment aged 0–15 years against the long-term ill in that population graded by sex was plotted.

Moving from the census back to the actual practice population, a practice profile of selected morbidity indicators was developed. It was possible to focus on a particular catchment of the population to study ischaemic heart disease morbidity (Figure 10).

Further mapping of the practice is underway which is exploring the following categories:

- Practice morbidity by age-sex
- Consultation rates for selected conditions
- Consultation rates by condition/age
- Occupation of patients
- Morbidity by occupation/unemployment
- Deaths by condition and place
- Emergency calls
- Prescribing patterns.

Exploratory workload data collected suggest that consultation rates differ in the areas of Ballantrae, Barrhill and Colmonell. Colmonell has no surgery and the people in this area consult less. The focus group explored the reasons for this by interviewing a random sample of residents in the three areas.

The time taken to reach Ballantrae by bus emerged as the major influence on attendance. The accessibility of the surgery, which is located on a hill, also acts as a deterrent. One solution was to hold a branch surgery in Colmonell on a weekly basis.

Lessons learnt

- It is possible to extract clinical data and present it geographically.

- Though currently at an experimental stage, geographical information systems such as MapInfo, in combination with other software such as Microsoft Excel and EMIS, have considerable potential in the clarification of local health needs.

PATIENT-CENTRED APPROACHES

Need and behavioural change
(Stott and Pill, 1990)

Aim

To explore why some people are more ready to modify their health-related behaviour than others, why some people are more successful in maintaining any changes made, and what members of the primary health care team can best do to foster such changes.

Background

The practice is situated in the middle of a large estate of mixed council and private housing and serves approximately 70% of the total estate population. Working class mothers were studied for two reasons: (a) women with children are among the most frequent users of primary health care services; (b) mothers are key figures whose health and behaviour are as likely to influence the health of their families as themselves. Lessons learnt from an in-depth study of their attitudes to health promotion through interviews and other qualitative methods informed local service development.

Methods

The age-sex register of the practice was used as a sampling frame. The names of women who met the following criteria were listed: having at least one child under 16, aged between 25 and 40 years, and classified as social class 4 or 5. The total list size was 266, of whom 77% were successfully interviewed.

Results

The majority of women considered that it was appropriate for their general practitioner to give lifestyle advice on the specific topics of smoking, weight and alcohol problems.

Over 90% of women counselled about smoking or weight reported that they had not been surprised or annoyed by the intervention, but advice on exercise was less readily accepted.

Just over half the sample claimed to have made at least one health-related behavioural change during the last five years. Those who did so were younger, better educated and more likely to be buying their house. Diet and exercise were the topics most frequently mentioned, followed by changes in smoking and work status.

There was little evidence of a rational approach leading to change. A mixture of influences—immediate triggers (for example, money difficulties) and long-term factors (for example, the support of partners) was invoked. The women were adapting to a variety of pressures and any action had to be seen in this context.

Lessons learnt

- Needs assessment may require painstaking investigative techniques. This project illustrates the blurred boundary between some research and health needs assessment.

26

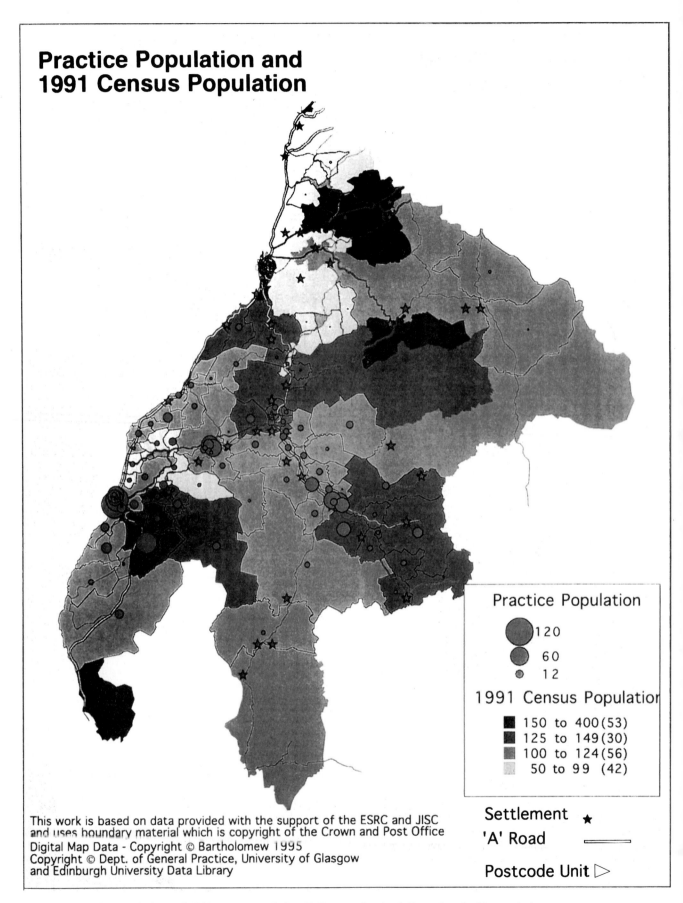

**Practice Population and
1991 Census Population**

Practice Population

120

60

12

1991 Census Population

150 to 400 (53)
125 to 149 (30)
100 to 124 (56)
50 to 99 (42)

Settlement ★
'A' Road ——
Postcode Unit ▷

Figure 9   Practice population and 1991 census population, Ballantrae, Scotland. Reproduced with permission.

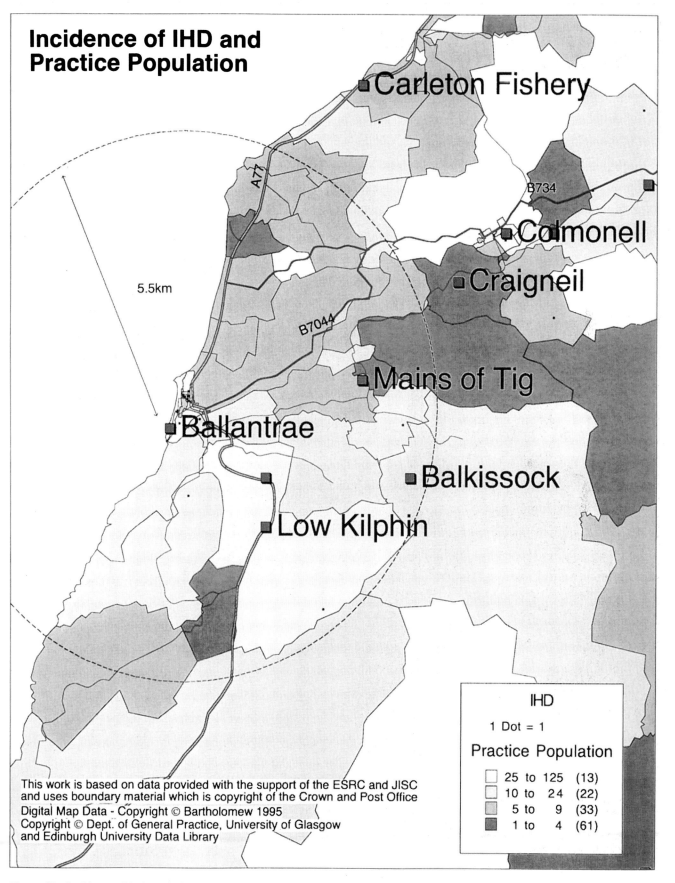

Figure 10 Incidence of ischaemic heart disease and practice population. Reproduced with permission.

- The patient is operating in a complex and demanding environment and health is often not the primary goal or consideration. Human behaviour can be explained by viewing the individual as engaged in meaningful interactions with other people and the environment.

- A fruitful relationship in health promotion is much more likely to develop where the person's priorities are established first and considered seriously before there is any attempt to encourage change. For example, the women studied placed greater health value on diet and nutrition whereas health professionals tend to place more emphasis on smoking and alcohol consumption.

From assessment to intervention: the role of a public health nurse
(Wearne, 1993)

Aim

To assess and meet needs in a deprived practice population using a step-wise approach:

- Community feedback on practice services

- The development of a comprehensive practice health profile by a public health nurse

- The categorization of needs identified

- The development of a health strategy

- The identification of resources to meet needs.

Background

Castlefields is a six-partner fundholding practice serving 12 300 people in Runcorn, an area of social deprivation. Situated in the centre of a large estate, Castlefields Health Centre is the only general practice in the area. The practice consists of six partners and a full complement of practice-based, community nursing and specialist staff.

The public health nurse (an ex-health visitor) was employed to work as a facilitator for the community helping people to express their health needs to the primary health care team. In turn, the nurse focused the team's attention on the services they delivered to explore the most effective and efficient way to meet the needs identified.

Methods

First, community feedback was obtained through regular meetings with local counsellors, a health forum, local residents and a survey of the practice population. This explored their views of various aspects of the services provided.

Secondly, practice profiling incorporated the results of a rapid appraisal exercise, census data, practice activity data and information from the local community trust. Causes of substantial mortality and morbidity among the practice population were identified. The public health nurse instigated a number of local community initiatives to address the identified needs. These included a cooking project, various keep fit initiatives, and a teenage health project.

Steps were taken to develop the profile as follows:

1. GETTING TO KNOW THE AREA

The public health nurse learnt about the history, geography and culture of the area by going out visiting and listening to the concerns of local groups and other agency workers.

Small group discussions and informal presentations were given to explain the project and to obtain feedback. This gave an indication of what it was like to live and work in the area and the community's strengths and weaknesses. It also helped to identify local leaders who were invaluable when setting up new initiatives.

2. IDENTIFYING INFORMATION SOURCES AND AREAS OF NEED

Basic information needs identified included:

- Mortality

- Morbidity

- Lifestyles

- Positive health

- Social characteristics and conditions

- Environmental factors

- Access and utilization of health care services

- Access and utilization of social services.

By seeking district, regional and national comparisons and exploring practice morbidity data, qualitative health data, social and environmental data, a wider picture of health in Castlefields was painted. The establishment of Castlefields Health Forum, a group of local people interested in the health and well-being of their community, also provided a means by which a more structured approach to obtaining information from local consumers of health care could be gained.

Castlefields profile took the following format:

- Introduction to the profile

- History/geography of the area

- The people

- Population data

- Birth data

- Infant mortality

- Adult mortality

- Positive health

- Lifestyle and risk factors

- Discussion

- Conclusions and recommendations.

The profile identified causes of substantial morbidity and mortality of those registered within the Castlefields practice and the ward. These were:

- Asthma

- Hypertension

- Diabetes

- Angina
- Bronchitis/emphysema
- Arthritis
- Mental health.

Based on available data and/or professional and local concerns, the profile identified many areas where there was scope for improvement:

- Environmental quality: (e.g. housing, lighting, dirt, and pollution)
- Economic investment
- Informed, planned parenthood
- Parental skills
- Dental health
- Diet (access, availability, skills)
- Reducing smoking
- Coping with stress
- Uptake of regular exercise
- Control of sexually transmitted disease
- Control of blood pressure
- Identifying the health needs of 15–24-year-olds
- Prevention of accidents and disabilities
- Improved access to maternity and child welfare services
- Rehabilitation facilities for people following operation, trauma, or illness
- Dignity and comfort at times of death.

3. CATEGORIZATION OF NEEDS IDENTIFIED

Quantitative data helped to give an indication of the size of the problem, allowed for comparisons, and helped to identify health needs. Qualitative data gave an indication of why there was a problem, emerging health concerns and the feasibility of local community health initiatives. The health needs identified were considered in relation to what was important and what could realistically be addressed. They were based, where possible, on the questions posed in Table 14.

Table 14 Importance and feasibility of addressing health needs

Importance
- Incidence and prevalence?
- Severity?
- Priority group?
- Cost to the community (financial and social)?
- Can it be viewed in a primary care context?
- Will prevention reduce future problems?

Feasibility
- Is this a community or professional issue?
- Is it preventable?
- Is community participation likely?
- Will inter-agency collaboration be forthcoming?
- Are there issues of equity?

- What resources will be required?
- Staff availability?
- Approachability?

Results

- A practice health strategy laid out a plan of action for each of the highlighted priorities. Each plan set aims and objectives with projected targets and outcomes to be achieved.

- By focusing on the needs of the area and how best to meet those needs, the team started to highlight priority areas of work and to question their own practice.

- For example, could activities traditionally done by a general practitioner be done by a nurse? A practice-based questionnaire highlighted the need for more appointments. This led to the recruitment of a nurse practitioner. Evaluation of this post has shown that this additional service is welcomed by patients.

- Many of the initiatives set up during the project were jointly supported by the local agencies involved. Closer working with other agencies provided opportunities to explore and use one another's networks for funding.

- Various projects were initiated, as described below.

1. YOUTH HEALTH INITIATIVE

This is a multidisciplinary venture, funded by Mersey Regional Health Authority for three years to explore the health needs of the young people in the area. A project co-ordinator has been appointed and the project aims to explore with young people their health needs and how best they should be met.

2. WHAT'S COOKING IN CASTLEFIELDS?

Initially a joint venture with the community centre run by the local authority. The aim was to establish a cookery course to explore how to obtain and maintain a healthy diet on a low budget. Initially aimed at young mothers the initiative has now been extended to include other target groups and is run through outside sponsorship.

3. NIFTY FIFTIES—AN EXERCISE CO-OP

Following a successful application for Look After Your Heart monies, an exercise co-op was set up with support from the local authority. This offers a health check and the opportunity to take part in activities and sports at a reduced cost and that would not normally be available e.g. horse riding, dry slope skiing.

4. VOLUNTEERS IN GENERAL PRACTICE

This was set up with the help of the local Runcorn Volunteer Bureau to improve the exchange of information between patients and the health centre. An information co-ordinator was co-opted to establish a library and to assist health promotion campaigns run in the practice.

5. HOUSING FOR HEALTH

This project is in the early stages of development. It is a joint venture with the local housing association to assess the health benefits gained from medical transfers.

Lessons learnt

- The health profile is a working tool and should be updated regularly (Table 15). It should be seen as belonging to all the people who live and work in the community and not to a single agency, profession or compiler. The profile is only the first step towards prioritizing and devising measurable objectives. It provides the baseline needs assessment from which new initiatives can be developed.

Table 15 The aims of a community health profile

- To give an insight into the nature and characteristics of a community
- To determine current effectiveness in relation to illness and the promotion of health
- To identify gaps in service
- To identify where new services are necessary to remove existing health inequity
- To recognize environmental changes that may be necessary to improve health
- To recognize and evaluate the need for inter-agency collaboration in meeting health needs
- To recognize and evaluate the need for community development

- Primary care nurses with public health skills have a valuable part to play in co-ordinating practice-based needs assessment. This role could include database establishment, community development, primary health care team education, local research and audit. Health visitors are often well equipped for this role.

- Baseline needs assessment is essential in developing service agreements and quality standards with other local providers. The involvement of patients is essential.

- It is important to recognize the untapped resources within the community. Many people freely gave their time for initiatives such as the Castlefields Health Forum and Volunteers in General Practice.

- Well-developed audit systems are inseparable from effective needs assessment. The Castlefields practice seeks evidence of the use of protocols and audit from all its providers. Fundholders are well placed to ensure their providers' practice is evidence based.

- Needs analysis is a valuable prerequisite to shifting care from the secondary sector. Fundholders can allocate resources to meet identified health needs.

A SYNTHESIS

A study of the use of four methods in a small neighbourhood
(Murray and Graham, 1995)

Aim

Much needs assessment work has been done in individual disciplines using single methods. Different approaches need to be used to create an overall picture. This work examined which approaches were most informative for which purposes.

Background

The setting for the study was Dumbiedykes, a small postwar council estate of 670 households in central Edinburgh. Four complementary approaches to health needs assessment were applied within a small neighbourhood. Each method was applied using resources which might be available to individual practices.

Methods

1. RAPID PARTICIPATORY APPRAISAL

A multi-sectoral team comprising a local general practitioner, health visitor, two social workers, and community education worker collected data from three sources:

- Existing documents about the neighbourhood

- Interviews with a range of informants

- Direct observations about the neighbourhood.

A profile was built using information collected on nine aspects of the community. These were brought together to form the information pyramid as described in Chapter 3. A semi-structured interview questionnaire was designed (see Appendix 3). Key informants in the study included people with professional knowledge about the community, community leaders and people who were centrally placed because of their work. Seventeen residents of Dumbiedykes were also selected to represent various age groups, social situations and health problems (Table 16). Several group interviews were carried out. Subsequently two focus groups were set up to discuss and allot priority to the problems identified and to explore potential interventions. The process took the team three months, spending four hours per week. Useful training material was available from WHO (Annett and Rifkin, 1995).

2. POSTAL SURVEY

A computer search was run using the General Practice Administration Scheme for Scotland (GPASS) software listing patients of the researchers' practice who were aged over 16 years and lived in Dumbiedykes. An output file was made and used with a mailmerge facility to address and send the questionnaires. Of the 993 residents of Dumbiedykes aged over 16 years (1991 census), 435 were registered at the study practice and all were surveyed. A questionnaire and a reply-paid envelope was posted with a letter signed by the senior partner explaining confidentiality and giving brief details of the proposed survey. Four weeks later a reminder with a fresh questionnaire was sent to non-respondents. Answers to

Table 16 List of key informants in Dumbiedykes participative appraisal

1. Voluntary worker, St Ann's Community Centre
2. Visiting sister, St Patrick's RC Church
3. Home care organizer, Social Work Department
4. Project director, South Side Care Project
5. Dumbiedykes Social Club Convenor
6. Local Lothian regional counsellor
7. Project co-ordinator, Safer Edinburgh Project
8. District counsellor
9. Local community involvement policeman
10. Receptionist, Mackenzie Medical Centre

11. Community development worker
12. Old Town Renewal Trust
13. Housing department officer, Edinburgh District Council
14. Pharmacist
15. Local district nurse
16. Head teacher and deputy head teacher, local primary school
17. Volunteer, Women's Royal Voluntary Service
18. Community psychiatric nurse, community drug problems service
19. Shopkeeper, Dumbiedykes store
20. Project co-ordinator, local youth project
21. Local health visitor
22. Public Transport Unit, Planning Department, Lothian Regional Council
23. Co-ordinator, Dumbiedykes Children's Centre
24. Recently retired local general practitioner
25. Group interview—South Side Care, Project Board of Directors
26. Group interview—Reminiscence Group
27. Group interview—Dumbiedykes Residents Association
28. Group discussion—teenage girls at youth project

open-ended questions were also considered together with the quantitative findings. A mixture of lay concepts and medical diagnoses were used. The survey covered:

- Chronic illness—a number of marker conditions which represent substantial areas of work in primary care were included

- Acute illnesses and experience of common symptoms

- Health status—the Nottingham Health Profile, a standard multidimensional measure based on lay concepts to assess both functional and emotional distress using six sub-scales was included

- Use of health services over six months

- Perceived need for current and potential services— respondents were asked how helpful a list of services or kinds of help would be to them personally

- Social and demographic characteristics of respondents

- People with long-term health problems; smokers and carers were asked further specific questions.

3. ROUTINELY AVAILABLE LOCAL STATISTICS

Lothian Health Information and Statistics Unit provided hospital-based morbidity information collected by the Scottish Morbidity Record (SMR) scheme relating to the 19 post codes for Dumbiedykes (population 1185) and for Lothian as a whole (population 726 010) for comparison. Inpatient and outpatient data were available at individual hospital episode level. The ninth revision of the International Classification of Diseases (ICD9) was used to decode diagnoses and the fourth revision of the Office of Population Censuses and Surveys, Classifications of Operations (OPCS 4) to decode operations and procedures. Complete data for 1991 were available. Data on births and deaths from the Registrar General for 1991 were also analysed. The 1991 census data were interrogated for the 19 postcodes that comprised Dumbiedykes.

4. PRACTICE-HELD INFORMATION

Information was obtained on the 538 residents of Dumbiedykes registered with the study practice using the following methods:

- From computerized records, the prevalence of chronic illness, repeat prescribing details, and various screening and health promotion data were obtained to give an overall medical profile.

- A random sample of 100 medical records was analysed. The incidence of acute illness, acute prescribing and psychosocial problems were recorded.

- Referrals of Dumbiedykes residents to hospitals and other agencies were examined for the previous year (1993–94).

- Deaths in Dumbiedykes from 1991–94 were reviewed.

- Data about surgery consultations, house calls, and out-of-hours visits to Dumbiedykes patients were extracted for the previous year (1993–94).

- The registers of drug addicts and HIV patients were examined.

- Data about Dumbiedykes patients were requested from the practice-attached health visitor, district nurse and the practice nurse.

Results

The data obtained were tabulated under the following headings: chronic medical conditions, acute illnesses and symptoms, behavioural factors, health status, health services, and the wider factors that influence health. Table 17 contains details of the main findings by method. For each condition, data are available from three or four sources, which allows for triangulation.

Table 18 shows that the prevalence of illness as found by postal survey was approximately twice that recorded in practice records.

Lessons learnt

- Rapid participatory appraisal encouraged a broad multidisciplinary approach to assessing health need (Murray, 1995). The role of selected users, community leaders and workers in prioritizing and planning care was developed. A neighbourhood profile was generated which detailed needs and available resources, and contained suggestions for change. The process in itself facilitated change. Few quantitative data were obtained. Co-ordinating the team was logistically difficult, and the work was time-consuming. Because people's broad priorities were heard, health service interventions were weighed against other options to improve the quality of life locally.

- The postal survey yielded detailed information about acute and chronic illness, and perceived need for existing and potential services for both users and non-users. The instrument could be re-applied to the same population or to a different population for comparisons over time or across areas. Individual community members identified their own needs. However, respondents were less likely to raise their own agendas and

Table 17 Data relating to specific medical and social factors according to the sources of information—practice data, local statistics, postal survey and rapid appraisal

	Practice data	Local statistics	Postal survey	Rapid appraisal
Chronic medical conditions				
Arthritis	Prevalence 12% 2% of males and 7% of females prescribed analgesics NSAIDs expensive prescribing costs Much loss of work	42% of residents over 50 years (30% in Lothian), 18% of outpatient referrals for orthopaedic surgery	31% prevalence Nottingham Health Profile revealed much pain and lack of mobility in over-65-year-olds 29% would find physiotherapy helpful 50% interested in alternative therapy	Arthritis restricted mobility in the elderly, accentuated by steep slopes and steps. Bus service that entered the estate, closer shops, more home helps, home delivery of medications by chemist, and more activities in the community rooms were suggested
Gastro-intestinal problems	12% prevalence 3.3% receiving H2 antagonist, gastro-intestinal system is the system with the highest prescribing costs	Endoscopy most common procedure in Lothian (second in Dumbiedykes) Abdominal pain second most common discharge diagnosis for Dumbiedykes and Lothian	18% of adults had experienced recurrent stomach problems in previous 6 months: constipation 15% diarrhoea or vomiting 13% poor appetite 13% 62% advice about healthy eating helpful 62% advice about losing weight helpful	Poor diet and eating habits identified locally. Local shop expensive and residents rarely bought fresh fruit and vegetables
Asthma/chronic bronchitis	6.5% prevalence 6% on bronchodilators 3% on inhaled steroids	Few outpatient referrals 13% of all admissions 3 deaths	14% prevalence 9% seen doctor in last 6 months for this	"Many toiling for breath" Damp housing causes asthma in children
Ischaemic heart disease (IHD)	Commonest cause of death 3.5% prevalence 3% on anti-platelet therapy 50% smokers	Commonest cause of deaths (Registrar General) Commonest discharge diagnosis in Dumbiedykes and Lothian Non-ischaemic chest pain eighth most common discharge diagnosis	10% perceived prevalence of heart problems/angina 72% requested advice about preventing heart disease 10% wanted more advice about healthy eating	IHD recognized as a major health problem "Anyone could have a heart attack" "Angina attacks" were caused by the steep hills
Hypertension	3.2% prevalence		13% stated they had "high blood pressure" 28% over-65-year-olds had "high blood pressure" 57% would find advice about their blood pressure helpful	
Acute illnesses				
Acute illnesses and symptoms	Percentage of Dumbiedykes patients who had consulted during the previous year: Urinary tract infection 32% (30%) Dermatological 34% (15%) Musculoskeletal 27% (12%) Minor trauma 5% (10%) Psychiatric 12% (10%) Gastro-intestinal 19% (8%) "Symptoms" 11% (16%) National averages are given in brackets (Fry, 1993)	In 14% of hospital admissions no definitive diagnosis made	Most common symptoms in the previous 6 months were: Cold/flu 46% Feeling tired 44% Headache 28% Difficulty sleeping 28% Patients experienced such symptoms twice as often as they attended the doctor or nurse for them. Although the incidence of skin problems (21%) and chronic cough (18%) was less, patients appeared to seek medical help more frequently when such problems arose	

Table 17 continued

	Practice data	Local statistics	Postal survey	Rapid appraisal
Behavioural factors				
Stress/depression	12% (medical records search) Medical records of 100 non-respondents to the postal survey reported stress/depression in 20, drug misuse in 8 and alcohol problems in 6	Census revealed many potential stressers: High unemployment Many single parents	18% prevalence of being anxious/depressed/bad nerves 10% seen doctor in the last 6 months for this 72% requested help or advice 16–44 age group scored highly on Nottingham Health Profile on emotional reaction and isolation sub-scales A help-line with someone who will listen to you was suggested	Stressful environment and lifestyles Regular citizen's advice, a course about alternative therapies, and a crèche were suggested
Smoking	50% current smokers Many smokers had died of smoking-related diseases	Frequent admissions for disorders of the circulatory and respiratory systems High smoking-related mortality	47% current smokers 50% of smokers want help or advice about giving up Opportunistic advice the most popular method of health promotion	Smoking a perceived cause of ill health in the community but a necessary coping mechanism or just a habit More young girls smoke 30% of the local shop's turnover was for cigarettes
Alcohol	13% of adults drink more than the recommended limit, 61% did not exceed and in 26% drinking status was not documented Socially isolated patients were at risk to drink to excess		8% remembered discussing alcohol with general practitioner in previous 6 months Help or advice about alcohol would be a great (10%) or some (22%) help	Alcohol a substantial but not an increasing problem. Some home helps considered that elderly clients drank to excess
HIV/drugs	Many patients on methadone substitution therapy lived in Dumbiedykes High turnover of drug addicts Several children with needlestick injuries Moving out of Dumbiedykes was the solution some patients gave for their drug problem	HIV carrier the fifth most common reason for adult hospital admission in 1991 Many indicators of socio-economic disadvantage revealed by census	6% wanted help or advice about illegal drugs 26% wanted help or advice about HIV "Would like HIV test without documentation"—freetext	Interviews revealed a broad and detailed picture. Some young families and socially isolated single parents were abusing drugs Drug users received prescribed substitutes and also bought extra medication from suppliers within Dumbiedykes Drug users were not concerned about HIV infection and even the few who still injected were not using condoms Most residents old and young alike knew of drug users and many commented: "This used to be a really nice area" Needles found by residents in bin stores
Reproductive health	Contraceptive prevalence rate over 50% Cervical smear screening rate 91% No home deliveries requested Breast feeding very rare	Suction termination of pregnancy most common operation in Lothian (2250 in 1991) Three mid-trimester therapeutic abortions were included in the 22 obstetric admissions from Dumbiedykes Single mothers accounted for 41% of admissions (25% in Lothian)	50% of females suffer period problems Menopause problems also common 80% of females would find cervical screening information helpful 82% of women requested information about breast screening 26% of males and females would value advice about HIV and AIDS	A focus group of young girls commented that they like to go along for the Pill with a friend Drug users admitted they rarely practise "safe sex"

Table 17 continued

	Practice data	Local statistics	Postal survey	Rapid appraisal
Health status Health status	Data which might suggest a low health status included: High prevalence of smoking, drinking and drug abuse Deprivation payments High consultation rates Dumbiedykes address	Ageing population with many indicators of socio-economic deprivation Dumbiedykes included in two postal sectors with deprivation categories of 4 and 5 (Carstairs)	High scores on all 6 Nottingham Health Profile sub-scales, especially for energy, pain and physical mobility Over-65 year olds scored highly on pain and physical mobility sub-scales 16–44 age groups scored highly on emotional reaction and social isolation sub-scales Residents scored their health as follows: excellent 10%, good 46%, fair 33%, poor/very poor 11% A female resident wrote: "I am crippled with knees but I'm in good health"	
Health services Use of health services	A high annual doctor/patient consultation rate of 5.1 and a total PHCT/patient rate of 7.3 Patients of the researcher's practice from more privileged areas consulted less, especially for out-of-hours calls Annual hospital referral rate was 400/1000, but the most common "referral letter" was to the district council requesting more suitable housing	Information from the Health Board revealed 87 general practitioners representing 42 partnerships had patients registered in Dumbiedykes; 25% of residents had general practitioners (and community nurses) based outwith the immediate area There was no evidence of an increased use of hospital services compared to Lothian	91% of respondents could consult a doctor on the same or the following day for an urgent problem; 13% reported home visits during the day and 14% reported out-of-hours call in the previous 6 months; reported out-of-hours telephone calls and visits (6pm–8am) were both double the actual practice average; an association was found between consultation rate and sex, presence of chronic disease and high Nottingham Health Profile scores; the doctor and the chiropodist were the health service workers most regularly visited; 78% requested more time to talk with the doctor during consultations; in the previous 6 months 13% had been admitted to hospital, and 13% had attended an accident and emergency department; 16% regularly attended an outpatient department	Appraisal yielded many constructive comments about the health services: telephone difficulties; delays in waiting for the doctor; some doctors are good listeners; lack of privacy at reception, long waiting times for occupational therapy and chiropody, shortage of district nurses, longer queues at the accident and emergency department and worse hospital discharge arrangements
Use of medicines	27% of Dumbiedykes residents received repeat prescriptions; the most commonly prescribed drugs were bronchodilators (6%), analgesics (4%), H2 blockers (3.3%) and inhaled steroids (3.2%). Analgesics, loop diuretics and ace-inhibitors were prescribed more frequently for Dumbiedykes residents than for the rest of the practice population. An average of 3.5 acute prescriptions were written per patient per year, 1.0 for antibiotics	The Scottish Prescribing Analysis reported that the practice was 3% above the Lothian average prescribing costs but 9% below the rest of Scotland	46% of respondents claimed they were on regular prescriptions (74% of over 64 year olds); 36% had bought medication, and 28% had bought vitamins or minerals; 16% had taken tranquillizers, antidepressants or hypnotics in the previous 6 months; only 3% had been given an unnecessary prescription; 9% had found prescription costs a problem; 62% requested an opportunity to discuss side effects of medication	The local chemist reported difficulties with drug users and that other patients were abusing anti-tussives and methanol. Some patients thought that the practice repeat prescribing system could be improved, and elderly patients requested chemists to deliver medication

Table 17 continued

	Practice data	Local statistics	Postal survey	Rapid appraisal
Health services—contd Consumer perceptions of local and national policies				Informants of the appraisal had little knowledge about the Patient's Charter and the community care plan
				Recent health policy interventions were thought by many to be cost cutting exercises
				Earlier hospital discharges resulted in more work for relatives, carers and district nurses
				Increasing care of people with serious mental illness in the community caused particular concern to neighbours, relatives and the local housing department
				The recent policy commitment by the NHS to "listen to local voices" was not perceived to be working by the local people
Wider factors that influence health Community composition		In 1991 there were fewer than half the number of children and over twice the number of pensioners than in 1974; only 3.4% had an ethnic background		Preponderance of elderly people and a considerable number of single people
		42% of Dumbiedykes residents compared to 30% in Lothian were aged 50 years or over		Newcomers to the area frequently had medical or social problems, and tended to be younger
				Little sense of community identity: "People don't seem to care," said a young mother
				Little opportunity to meet except on the lifts or waiting for a bus
				Only 31% were married, and 36% lived alone
Physical environment				The hills in and out of the estate, the numerous steps, and the generally poor access featured as major issues. Lack of play areas for toddlers and young children frequently mentioned
				Dog fouling was a greater issue than vandalism or violence
				Apart from one small expensive general store, all shopping, surgeries and other services were up steep hills
				Residents reported problems with poorly fitting windows, lack of insulation, damp bedrooms and difficulties with heating
				Many initiatives to address the difficult physical environment were suggested: improve the local bus service, inform all residents about Dial-a-bus, taxi-cards,

Table 17 continued

	Practice data	Local statistics	Postal survey	Rapid appraisal
Wider factors that influence health—contd Physical environment—contd				and Handi-cabs, and regular housing advice to be made available in the community room
Community organization and capacity for change				Compared to the pre-war period there were very few services in Dumbiedykes
				Most informants identified a named volunteer worker and her community centre colleagues, as being the main community activists
				A local counsellor commented on the lack of a "heart" or "centre" in the scheme
				Three house groups run by a nearby church gave social and spiritual support to some residents
				The residents' association was not well known and the younger age groups were poorly represented
Socio-economic environment		26% of males and 11% of females were recorded as unemployed in the 1991 census Moreover 44% of the 16 to 19-year-olds and 37% of the 20 to 40-year-old males were unemployed 20% owned housing compared to 60% in Lothian 15% of households owned a car compared to 42% in Lothian	House ownership was 34%, car ownership 25% Residents' most common worries were lack of money (28%), housing (20%), relationship with partner (18%), and work (16%)	Many residents found it hard to manage financially, especially the elderly, people on benefits, and those who did not quite qualify for benefits. Although 80% of houses had central heating, few used it as it was electric only and very expensive. The local pharmacist estimated that 90% of prescriptions were exempt and the local head mistress estimated that 80% of children received free school meals. The housing department reported a number of residents in rent arrears and the youth project subsidized a number of children for their activities. The career service reported a dearth of work opportunities
Social services				The local social services were well known, well used and appreciated. However, the non-locally-based services were little known and a wish for more information was expressed. A typical comment was: "It's finding out about them that's the difficulty." Most knew of some services but not how to use them. More effective publicity to bridge the information gap was suggested. The home help service was considered to be under-resourced. Some voluntary agencies were underutilized

Table 18 Comparison of prevalences of conditions and social factors by method

	Routine statistics %	Postal survey %	Practice data %
Arthritis		31	12
Stomach problems		20	12
Stress/depression		18	12
Asthma/chronic bronchitis		14	6.5
Hypertension		13	3.2
Heart disease/angina		10	3.5
URTI (last 6 months)		46	20
Limiting long-term illness	20	22	17
Repeat prescriptions		46	27
House ownership	20	34	
Car ownership	15	25	
Telephone		81	67

there was a low response rate in young men. Considerable time, resources and specific skills were again required.

- Routine local statistics gave a descriptive account of morbidity and socio-economic indicators and allowed comparison with regional norms. Collaboration between public health and primary care allowed sharing of perspectives and skills, and permitted comparison of ward-based and practice-based datasets.

- Practice data collection facilitated teamwork. Much information was available from computerized data, medical records, annual reports and financial statements but this had to be analysed and 'cleaned'. Much local knowledge of the neighbourhood was implicit, and was explicitly documented with some effort.

- The participatory appraisal was the only method which brought about change during the data collection process itself. Subsequent to the participatory appraisal, many of those responsible for non-health services have responded to suggestions from the community. The local bus route has been altered to run into the council estate resulting in a 30% increase in passengers. The district council housing department has provided fenced-off play areas. The community room is now used by district and regional counsellors, community education classes, and two residents' associations. Three companies are tendering to construct a local supermarket. Many practical suggestions for improving local medical facilities were also made and have been acted on; a second telephone line has been installed in the doctors' surgery, there are toys in the surgery play area, patients are addressed in a fashion more acceptable to them, and a ramp is to be provided. The potential of the other methods to cause change was not tested. It may be that changes will happen on a longer timescale.

- Different methods yielded complementary insights into health needs generally, and into specific problems. With asthma/chronic bronchitis and ischaemic heart disease (examples of ongoing physical problems), practice data and survey data had the greatest utility. The problems of drug abuse and HIV in the community were best revealed by rapid appraisal and

data collection within the practice, a combination also found useful to explore other psychosocial issues. The postal survey usefully supplemented practice data about acute illness within the community. Inpatient admissions compared with the rest of Lothian provided a proxy of need for secondary care. The postal survey was able to display a different frequency of perceived and formally diagnosed illness. Health service planning was best informed by the appraisal and census data. Indeed a more immediate need for "non-health" services was articulated by the appraisal. A subjective indication of the utility of the methods to yield information about specific issues in this study is given in Table 19.

Table 19 A subjective indication of the utility of the methods to yield information about specific issues in this study

	Practice data	Local statistics	Postal survey	Rapid appraisal
Chronic medical conditions				
Arthritis	2	3	2	2
Gastro-intestinal	2	3	2	3
COAD	1	3	2	4
IHD	2	3	2	3
Hypertension	1	4	2	4
Acute illnesses				
Acute illness	2	4	1	3
Behavioural factors				
Stress/depression	3	4	2	2
Alcohol	2	4	3	2
Smoking	3	4	2	2
Drug abuse/HIV	2	3	4	1
Reproductive health	2	2	2	2
Health status				
Health status	2	3	1	3
Health services				
Use of health services:				
Primary	1	4	2	2
Secondary	2	1	3	3
Use of medicines	2	1	3	3
Wider factors that influence health				
Community composition	3	2	3	3
Physical environment	2		4	1
Capacity for change	3		3	1
Socio-economic	3	2	2	1
Context of service provision	4	2	3	1
Consumer perception	3	4	2	1
Public involvement				

Key: 1. Method very informative about this issue.
    4. Method yields little information about this issue.

- Community involvement is important, both as a democratic goal in itself and as a potentially useful means of achieving improvements in health. The extent of public involvement in these methods, in decreasing order, was: rapid appraisal (where providers and patients interacted and learnt from each other); postal survey (when respondents' perceptions and suggestions were read and analysed); practice data gathered by a team in daily contact with patients over many years; and routine statistics supplied without any patient involvement.

SUMMARY

This chapter has illustrated several examples of different approaches to data collection as a basis for needs assessment. They illustrate several points:

- The myriad of different possible approaches to needs assessment in practice

- The close relationship of needs assessment to practice profiling (page 28), evaluation (page 17), audit (page 20) and even research (pages 24, 25).

- Overlaps between practice-based, patient-centred and public health-led approaches (pages 22, 30).

- The essence of needs assessment is its impact on subsequent decision-making and whether it produces changes (pages 24, 28).

- The scope for harnessing new technologies in this area (pages 24).

- The value of triangulating approaches (pages 22, 30).

A practical approach to reconciling the different choices available is suggested in the final chapter.

CHAPTER 5
Ways forward

THE separation of purchaser from provider of health services looks set to remain for the foreseeable future (Ham and Shapiro, 1995). General practitioners' critical position as both purchasers and providers gives them great influence. This influence will be at the cost of ever-increasing accountability for the budgets that they control. This will mean continuing pressure to undertake and participate in needs assessment activities. However, these activities have opportunity costs. It is not yet clear how best to organize practices to fulfil these functions. It is unlikely that all doctors need to devote time to them. Growing specialization within general practice makes it more likely that these tasks will be divided among those with special interests.

Other obstacles are summarized in the first part of this chapter. Ways of optimizing the impact of needs assessment are then discussed. Finally, for those seeking a path through the maze of available options, a staged approach is described in conclusion.

Challenges

Problems likely to be encountered when promoting a practice-based approach to needs assessment are as follows:

Ethical

The traditionally individualistic approach of general practitioners may be difficult to reconcile with the utilitarian approach to planning at more central level.

Recent contractual changes have promoted a population-oriented approach in general practice, for example through target setting for cervical cytology, immunization and health promotion. There is no evidence that patients prefer doctors to devolve responsibility for resource allocation to managers.

Skills shortages

Epidemiological and data-handling skills are in short supply in primary care. There are insufficient numbers of public health doctors to allow dedicated support to all practices. Educational strategies are needed to address these shortages.

The time and resources required can be exaggerated. Basic numeracy and common sense are the most important prerequisites.

Lack of incentives

The health promotion banding and chronic disease management arrangements provided some incentive to explore the practice population's needs in relation to these diseases. There are few other inducements to take on the extra work implied.

Incentives should be developed in future. Local medical committees are to approve health promotion priorities from October 1996. Health authorities may be given discretion to set other targets in conjunction with primary health care teams should the national contract be dis-

mantled. Increasingly, general practitioners will be required to justify bids for resources (for example, staffing allocations) in terms of locally-identified needs.

Methodological

The absence of common disease definitions, common classification systems and compatible software, and the partial recording of practice activity will limit the value of practice databases to health authorities/boards in the near future. The difficulty of interpreting referral rates or prescribing data underline the dangers of using measures of practice activity as indices of need.

The widening use of Read codes and the development of interactive software systems will increase commonality in future. Several general practice networks are now sharing and auditing morbidity data between practices (see Chapter 4).

Compartmentalization

Assessment of health care needs is integrally related to service evaluation. Many of the activities described above fall within a broad definition of audit.

Many medical audit advisory groups (MAAGs or their successors) are using *Health of the Nation* priorities to frame their agendas for the coming year. Health authorities and medical audit advisory groups share an interest in focusing audit activity on identified practice priorities.

Tension between practice and health authority/board priorities

Rigid imposition of nationally determined health promotion priorities stifled local innovation.

Allowing practices increasing autonomy to set their own objectives in the light of identified needs will result in greater commitment to achieving those objectives. The health promotion scheme is being developed along these lines.

Professional isolation

A practice-based approach to needs assessment can overlook the enormous volume of information collected by and for community units. Primary health care teams may centre on neighbourhoods. Health visitors' skills in this area are easily overlooked.

Meeting as a practice team to define practice population needs systematically can be an important team-building exercise in its own right. It may be the first time that all members of the primary health care team have fully appreciated other members' roles, skills and contributions.

Relevance of information

Much of the most easily available data are ward based and of doubtful value for practices.

Mapping packages are now available that allow the calculation of more practice-specific markers of need, such as practice deprivation scores. Practices need to know how representative their patient population is in terms of age and sex of the wards in which they live.

Rationing

Encouraging needs assessment activity may lead to increased demands on limited resources and generate unfulfillable expectations. We know little about how the public prioritize treatments (Honigsbaum et al., 1995).

Full assessment of needs heightens understanding about the effectiveness of different health care interventions and the need to prioritize. Practitioners are daily engaged in implicit rationing and are well aware of the finite nature of health service resources. Without this fuller understanding, a primary health care team is less likely to make the changes in one area that will offset new demands in another.

Decision-making must be systematic and explicit if it is to be defended to patients and their representatives. There is growing literature on the public's views suggesting, for example, that they tend to accord a higher priority to treatments for younger rather than older people and particularly to lifesaving treatments (Bowling, 1996). Finally, it is not self-evident that with better information patients will generate infinite demands (Frankel, 1992).

Lack of evidence

The literature available to inform needs assessment is limited and much of it focuses on secondary care. Few diseases have been adequately researched and this is especially true of outcome studies in the primary health care setting where many of the outcomes may be emotional or subjective in nature and where few outcome measures have been validated.

The importance of critical appraisal skills is increasingly recognized. The science of systematic review is underpinning a revolution in the nature of information exchange. The emergence of the Cochrane Collaboration has opened up new frontiers for those promoting evidence-based medicine.

Organizational uncertainty

No-one can confidently predict the future of purchasing. A sense of the ephemeral nature of today's organizational structures undermines commitment to tasks that may be seen as 'managerial'.

The desire to influence the way resources are allocated will survive political changes. The NHS is to be 'primary care led' for the foreseeable future. The responsibility of the profession is to ensure their new powers are used to the greater good of the patients they serve.

Nature of accountability

In assuming direct control over public monies fundholders take on responsibilities for engaging their practice population in the process of allocating resources. The same ethical imperative faces health authorities. The frameworks for holding them to account are at an early stage of development. However, increasingly all general practices are likely to be subject to similar monitoring.

Formal mechanisms for holding doctors to account for the money they spend are inescapable. Constructive dialogue is possible where health boards/commissions approach this process with sensitivity.

Conceptual

Some of the approaches described imply fundamental reappraisal of the health professional's role and the balance of power within the doctor-patient relationship. This is threatening.

The National Health Service is only a mirror for social changes taking place across the public sector where the consumer's contribution to service planning is growing. Work beyond the surgery door can be a source of enormous professional satisfaction as well as yielding significant health benefits for patients.

The greatest obstacle is lack of time. Such work has opportunity costs. Little is known of the cost-effectiveness of the different approaches described. Further research is necessary to develop and test models of health needs assessment.

Effecting change

There are three strands to the planning process. The first two were considered in Chapter 2. The third—describing how you are going to get there—is equally important. Needs assessment is futile if it does not result in improved services to patients. Chapter 4 illustrated how some teams moved forward having identified and prioritized needs. The results of needs assessment work therefore need to be encapsulated in a practice strategy or business plan. The clear definition of objectives, describing what needs to be done by whom and by when, is invaluable. Such documents can also be short. Objectives need to be appropriate, practical and timely. Without clear milestones for the achievement of constituent parts of the plan, timetables invariably slip. Regular review meetings are important for revisiting objectives and the use of resources. Plans can be distilled into single sheets such as a Gantt chart (Figure 11).

There is a large literature on the art of change management but little concerned directly with general practice (Pringle et al., 1991; Spiegel et al., 1992). The interested reader is referred to one of several general introductions (Plant, 1987; Open University, 1991).

The key to effecting change is an understanding of the opportunities that may facilitate and the obstacles that may obstruct what is being attempted—knowing which 'levers' to use. An understanding of the sources of finance, their planning cycles and the criteria used to fund projects is particularly important. A list of likely targets is included in Table 20.

Table 20 Possible funding sources

FHSAs/DHAs/health boards purchasing plans
Local authorities, e.g. joint finance
Primary care development monies
Audit funds
Research & Development budgets
Institutional grants/fellowships/bursaries
Training funds
Voluntary organizations

Health authorities/boards nowadays clearly indicate the timing of development bids and the structure of applications they wish practices to submit. There is little point in requesting new resources in April if purchasing plans

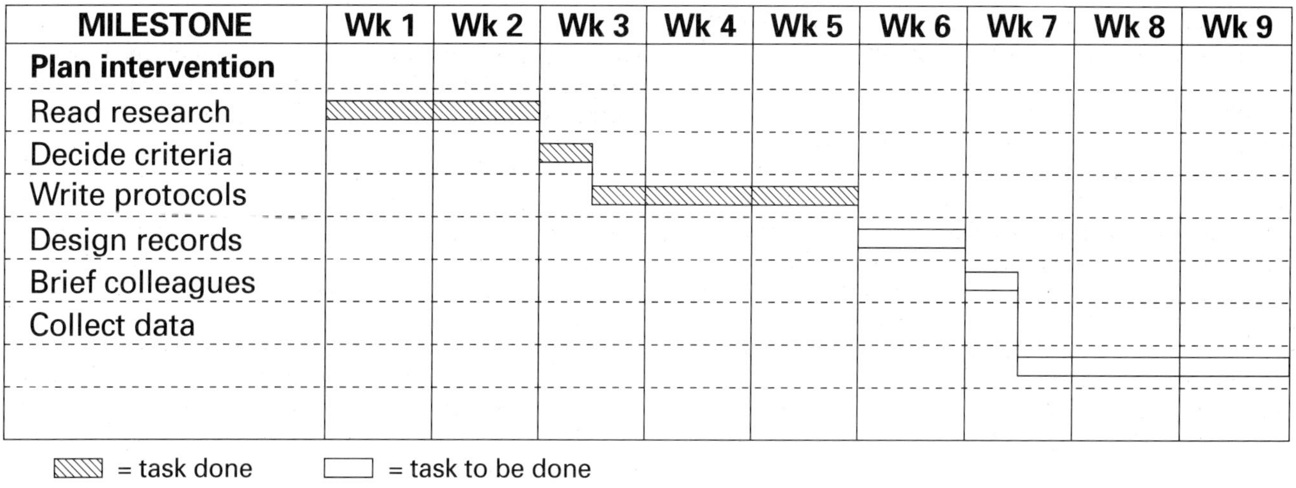

MILESTONE	Wk 1	Wk 2	Wk 3	Wk 4	Wk 5	Wk 6	Wk 7	Wk 8	Wk 9
Plan intervention									
Read research	▨	▨							
Decide criteria			▨						
Write protocols			▨	▨	▨				
Design records						☐			
Brief colleagues							☐		
Collect data							☐	☐	☐

▨ = task done   ☐ = task to be done

Figure 11   Sample Gantt chart

were finalized in March. That said, there is often more flexibility in the system than may be realized.

Finally, plans are more likely to be realized where they are 'owned'. For this reason, patient-centred approaches often result in more immediate changes (Chapter 4, page 25). Paradoxically, data rigorously quantified at a distance from the coalface may be less powerful than crude qualitative data in moving decision-makers. The importance of community participation has been repeatedly stressed in this document (Neve and Taylor, 1995). General practitioners are often unaware of the range of different agencies in the community that may assist them.

A composite model

A coherent, practical approach is required for needs assessment in general practice (Gillam, 1992b). Caution must be exercised when using only one method. Practice data may understate the prevalence of disease in the community. Postal surveys have to be interpreted carefully. Doctors and patients may ascribe different meanings to words such as 'hypertension'. A small number of in-depth interviews will not be representative of the study population. A few unusual events may skew small area statistics. Thus, different approaches to needs assessment are required to inform the commissioning process.

All methods incur considerable time and effort. They can be simplified with experience. A locally appropriate method-mix would seek data from various sources according to ease of access, potential utility and possible resources. A composite practice-based model starts with the practice team's knowledge and experience of working in the local community. It might involve:

- Collecting practice-based information (Table 3)

- Gathering other routinely available morbidity and census data with the assistance of the public health department (Table 21)

- Carrying out a participatory appraisal to identify areas of perceived health need (Table 16, Appendix 3)

- Conducting a survey to identify needs (Table 6)

- Preparing a practice profile and action plans

- Implementing and reviewing changes.

Table 21   Routinely available statistics

1. Inpatient data
- Ten most frequent diagnoses made at hospital discharge (rates per 1000 residents), both episode-based and case-linked data
- Admissions (rate per 1000 residents)
- Mean waiting time (males and females)
- Three most frequent operations/procedures (rates per 1000), both episode-based and case-linked data

2. Census
- Percentage of residents with limiting long-term illness
- Demographic profile, in 5-year bands
- Unemployment rates, male and female (%)
- Percentage house owners
- Percentage car owners
- Percentage of households with lone parents

3. Outpatient data
- Outpatient referral rate per 1000 residents
- Referral rates for three most frequent specialties
- Mean waiting times

4. Obstetric data
- Number of deliveries (rate per 1000 residents)
- Outcomes, including spontaneous and therapeutic abortions
- Single mothers (%)

Conclusion

The challenge for public health and primary care is to work together to address social and environmental causes of ill health and thereby to improve the health of populations. In 1883 Tennant-Gardner, the first Medical Officer of Health in Glasgow, warned of the danger of divorcing everyday clinical care from the population perspective. A century later we hear the same calls for general practitioners and public health physicians to rediscover their common roots and core values (Hannay, 1993). Collaboration in health needs assessment can strengthen these links while providing a powerful force for change in local communities.

APPENDIX 1
Useful resources

USEFUL ADDRESSES

1. NHS Centre for Reviews and Dissemination (NHSCRD)

NHS Centre for Reviews and Dissemination
University of York
York YO1 5DD
Tel: 01904 433634
Fax: 01904 433661
Email: revdis@uk.ac.york
http://www.york.ac.uk/inst/crd/info.htm

- The Centre was established to provide information on effectiveness of treatments and delivery of organization of health care (including effectiveness of health technologies).

- It undertakes and commissions rigorous reviews of research findings on effectiveness of health care (including those on health promotion interventions).

- It maintains databases of literature reviews and economic evaluations.

- A range of databases is available on-line and on disk:
  —*Database of Published Reviews*: An international register of good quality research reviews of the effectiveness of health care interventions. It is prospective and concentrates on interventions relevant to *Health of the Nation* and other selected topics.
  —*Database of Economic Evaluations*: A register of published economic evaluations of health care interventions. Records include structured summary and a quantitative assessment together with details of any practical implications for the NHS.
  —*Text database* of reviews undertaken by the Centre and other agencies it commissions. This includes full text of *Effective Health Care Bulletins*.

2. Cochrane Collaboration

The UK Cochrane Centre
NHS Research & Development Programme
Summertown Pavilion
Middle Way, Oxford OX2 7LG
Tel: 01865 516300
Fax: 01865 516311
Email: cochrane@vax.ox.ac.uk
http://hiru.mcmaster.ca/cochrane/default.htm

The Centre's role is to facilitate, maintain and disseminate systematic, up-to-date reviews of randomized controlled trials of health care. The Cochrane Library is available in medical libraries. It is regularly updated and includes the following:

- *Cochrane Pregnancy and Childbirth Database (CCPC)*: This consists of over 600 systematic, regularly updated reviews of randomized trials of care in pregnancy and childbirth.

- *Effective Care in Pregnancy and Childbirth and a Guide to Effective Care in Pregnancy and Childbirth*: Both books list (a) forms of care that have been shown to reduce negative outcomes; (b) forms of care that appear promising but require further evaluation; (c) forms of care with unknown effects; and (d) forms of care that are so unlikely to be of benefit that they should be abandoned.

- *Systematic Review Database (CDSR)*: The database incorporates material from three sources. These are:
  —*Cochrane Reviews*: reviews, protocols and titles submitted by registered Collaborative Review Groups.
  —*Bibliographies*: existing reports of systematic reviews, reviews assessed for quality by the NHSCRD, reviews on the database of the International Network of Agencies for Health Technology Assessment, and methodological articles.
  —*Cochrane Collaboration*: contains extensive information on contact details, review groups, methods groups, and Cochrane centres.

3. Wessex Institute of Public Health

Wessex Institute of Public Health
Dawn House
Highcroft
Romsey Road
Winchester SO22 5DH
Tel: 01962 863511

- Developed by the *Epidemiologically Based Needs Assessment Reviews* (commissioned by the Department of Health). Produced in two volumes, they review 20 important conditions and services which cover over one third of the "burden of disease" in most western countries. Topics covered include:
  —Diabetes mellitus
  —Renal disease
  —Stroke
  —Lower respiratory disease
  —Coronary heart disease
  —Colorectal cancer
  —Cancer of the lung
  —Total hip replacement
  —Total knee replacement
  —Cataract surgery
  —Hernia repair
  —Varicose vein treatments
  —Prostatectomy for benign prostatic hyperplasia
  —Mental illness
  —Dementia
  —Alcohol misuse
  —Drug misuse

—People with learning disabilities
—Community child health services
—Family planning, abortion and fertility services

- The Wessex Institute also undertakes *Health Technology Evaluation Research Reviews*. Two volumes covering a range of specialist interventions are currently available. Topics covered include:
—Magnetic resonance imaging in the diagnosis of multiple sclerosis
—Magnetic resonance imaging in the diagnosis of knee disorders
—Ceredase for Gaucher's disease
—Lithotripsy for gallstones
—Adult cochlear implants
—Anticoagulation for non-rheumatic atrial fibrillation
—Cardiac rehabilitation.

4. Nuffield Institute for Health

Nuffield Institute for Health
71–75 Clarendon Road
Leeds LS2 9PL
Tel: 01132 336633

- The Institute's aim is to improve expertise in health and social care policy. There are several specialist units focusing on such topics as community care, quality assurance, and public health. The Institute's information resource centre has a substantial library and provides a wide range of information through HELMIS (the Health Management Information Service).

5. UK Health Outcomes Clearing House

- The UK Health Outcomes Clearing House is based within the Nuffield Institute for Health (see above).

- It aims to collect, critically appraise, collate and disseminate the most up-to-date information on health assessment and health care outcomes. The outcomes activity database contains details of about 700 outcomes-related projects.

- Information is distributed freely through newsletters and update bulletins. It currently produces *Outcomes Briefing*. Other activities include:
—Acting as a resource centre for outcomes assessment materials
—Being a focal point for exchange of information on health services outcomes
—Reviewing collected measures and methods
—Providing an information and advisory service.

6. Yorkshire Collaborating Centre for Health Services Research

Yorkshire Collaborating Centre for Health Services Research
University of Leeds
Nuffield Institute for Health
71–75 Clarendon Road
Leeds LS2 9PL
Tel: 01132 336983

- The Centre acts as a provider of reviews and research. Reviews currently available include:
—NHS Purchasing Policy: a dilemma concerning a new treatment for multiple sclerosis
—Research into practice: policy options for NHS purchasing authorities
—Cochlear implant technology and NHS purchasing policy
—Complex, dual chamber, rate-responsive pacemaker: literature review.

7. MIQUEST

Software and training material are available from the Clinical Information Consultancy, 93 Wantage Road, Reading, Berkshire RG13 2SX. Tel: 01734 585954.

USEFUL PUBLICATIONS

1. Evidence-based Purchasing

A bi-monthly digest of evidence from the former South & West Region about effective care to support the commissioning role. It includes features and short reports on evidence of effectiveness of health interventions. Recent topics include:

- Maternity services
- Near-patient testing
- Organization of palliative care services
- Cochlear implant technology
- Shared care for diabetes.

2. Central Health Outcomes Unit

This is a joint policy/management executive unit within the Department of Health working on the development and application of health outcomes assessment.

Population Health Outcome Indicators for the NHS
(a) A feasibility study
(b) A consultation document

- Breast cancer
- Diabetes mellitus
- Peptic ulcer
- Osteoporosis and hip fracture
- Unplanned pregnancy
- Congenital abnormalities
- Skull fracture/intracranial injury
- Hypertension and stroke
- Perinatal and infant mortality
- Immunizations
- Early orchidopexy for cryptorchidism
- Acceptance rates/RRT
- Mental health indicators

- Tuberculosis
- Asthma
- Chronic rheumatic heart disease
- Hodgkin's disease
- Cancer of the cervix
- Maternal mortality

3. Medicines Resource Centre (MeRec)

- MeRec is funded by the Department of Health. It produces bulletins and briefings on medicinal productions and matter relating to prescribing practice.

4. Effective Health Care Bulletins

Tel: 01279 623924

These bulletins are based on a systematic review of literature on clinical effectiveness, cost-effectiveness and acceptability of health service interventions. The NHSCRD have published 11 bulletins. A further six are expected in 1996. Reviews on the following topics are currently available:

- Screening for osteoporosis to prevent fractures
- Stroke rehabilitation
- The management of subfertility
- The treatment of persistent glue ear in children
- The treatment of depression in primary care
- Cholesterol screening and treatment
- Brief interventions and alcohol use
- Implementing clinical guidelines
- Management of menorrhagia
- The prevention and treatment of pressure sores
- Benign prostatic hyperplasia.

5. Effectiveness Matters

This is an update on the effectiveness of important health care interventions.. It is produced by researchers at the NHSCRD. The first issue covered Aspirin and Myocardial Infarction and the second issue covered *Helicobacter pylori* and Peptic Ulcer.

6. Bandolier

Published by the Anglia and Oxford RHA Research & Development Unit, *Bandolier* newsletter is designed to keep purchasers up to date with both local and national initiatives, and literature on the effectiveness of health care interventions. This popular effectiveness bulletin is published monthly and is free to all general practitioners. http://www.jrz.ox.ac.UK/Bandolier

7. Health of the Nation Target Effectiveness Documents

- Target effectiveness and cost effectiveness guide for coronary heart disease and stroke.
- Target effectiveness guide for cervical cancer.

Health of the Nation Key Area Handbooks

- Coronary heart disease
- Cancers
- Mental illness
- Accidents
- HIV/AIDS and sexual health

8. Register of Cost-Effectiveness Studies

- The register contains details of almost 150 economic studies of health care interventions, covering most branches of medicine. The NHSCRD has been commissioned to make the register more user friendly.

9. ACP Journal Club/Evidence-Based Medicine

- Published bi-monthly by the American College of Physicians, *ACP Journal Club* details abstracts from published studies and reviews on important advances in treatment, diagnosis, cause, prognosis and the economics of internal medicine. A new journal (*Evidence-Based Medicine*), with a broader remit and a European focus, was launched in October 1995.

10. Clinical Standards Advisory Group

Tel: 0171 972 4918

- The Clinical Standards Advisory Group (CSAG) is a multiprofessional group that assesses clinical services against standards previously set by professional bodies. The reports of these groups can inform local peer review. CSAG reports include:
  —Stillbirths and deaths in infancy—access and availability of specialist services
  —Access to and availability of coronary artery bypass grafting and coronary angioplasty
  —Back pain
  —Childhood leukaemia, access to and availability of specialist services
  —Cystic fibrosis, access to and availability of specialist services
  —The epidemiology and cost of back pain
  —Neonatal intensive care, access to and availability of specialist services
  —Standards of care for people with diabetes
  —Urgent and emergency admissions
  —Women in normal labour
  —Schizophrenia.

11. Clinical Guidelines

The Department of Health offers a small portfolio of clinical guidelines from professional bodies that take account of the research evidence for best effective clinical practice. Guidelines commended in 1993 and 1994 are as follows:

- Radiology: Making the best use of a Department of Radiology

- Asthma: *Thorax* (1993); Guidelines on the Management of Asthma

- Diabetes: Recommendations for the Management of Diabetes in Primary Care

- Heart Disease: British Cardiac Society and the Royal College of Physicians. The investigation and management of stable angina

- Leg Ulcers: The management of leg ulcers in the community. University of Liverpool

- Neonatal Respiratory Distress: Development of audit measures and guidelines for good practice in the management of neonatal distress syndrome

- Head Injury: Report of the Working Party on Head Injuries (1986)

- Cancer: Guidelines for managing cancer pain

- Hospital Infection: Revised guidelines for the control of epidemic methicilin-resistant *Staph-Aureus*.

12. Agency for Health Care Policy Research Publications

This American Agency has a clearing house for effectiveness reports, clinical practice guidelines and other policy reports. Full-text versions of the clinical guidelines are available through the Internet.

- *Clinical Effectiveness in Allied Health Practices*: critical literature review (328 papers concerning the effec-

tiveness of treatment provided by physiotherapists, dietitians, and so on).

The following clinical practice guidelines are currently available:

- Acute pain management: operative or medical procedures trauma

- Urinary incontinence in adults

- Pressure ulcers in adults: prediction and prevention

- Cataract in adults: management of functional impairment

- Depression in primary care; Vol 1. Detection and diagnosis

- Depression in primary care; Vol 2. Treatment of major depression

- Sickle cell disease, screening, diagnosis, management and counselling in newborn and infants

- Evaluation and management of early HIV infection

- Benign prostatic hyperplasia: diagnosis and treatment

- Management of cancer pain

- Unstable angina: diagnosis and management

- Heart failure; management of patients with left ventricular systolic dysfunction

- Otitis media with effusion in young children

- Quality determinants of mammography

- Acute low back pain in adults

- Treatment of pressure ulcers

- Post stroke rehabilitation

- Cardiac rehabilitation.

APPENDIX 2

Public health data sources

D ATA sources comprise demographic data, activity data and health data. Their chief defect, as already mentioned, is that they are collected on (large) populations that are geographically defined. The 1991 census data can be disaggregated to post code level but do not strictly relate to practice populations. With careful interpretation, they are nonetheless useful ingredients for the practice population profile.

DEMOGRAPHIC DATA

Population data

The baseline population data, from which all other population data are derived, are the results of the decennial census. The district population and the age breakdown are contained in a book called *Census 1991— Key Statistics for Local Authorities* from the Office of Population Censuses and Surveys (OPCS, 1992).

Population estimates and projections

Population estimates refer to educated guesses of the population from the time of the last census to the present day, while population projections refer to educated guesses for the future. Population estimates are calculated by OPCS by taking the census data as a baseline, by using data on births and deaths since the time of the census and then estimating migration in and out of the district. Mid-year estimates of population are prepared because the census takes place only every 10 years. These figures are particularly useful in areas where rapid changes are taking place. (The address for OPCS is Titchfield, Fareham, Hampshire PO15 5RR.)

Social characteristics

Most information available on the social characteristics of the people comes from the census. *Census 1991* contains the following information for districts:

- Economic activity
- Industry of employment (10% sample)
- Travel to work (10% sample)
- Number of households/household size/economically active adults
- Households with children/one-adult households with children
- Ethnic group.

As regards electoral ward data, the following information may be obtained:

- Population of at least 65 years of age
- Elderly people living alone
- Population under five years of age

- Families that are one-parent families
- Workforce who are unskilled
- Workforce who are unemployed
- Households that lack basic amenities
- Population who were born in countries other than the UK
- People who consider they have a limiting long-term illness.

Deprivation indices

Several indices of deprivation have been developed over recent years, which are based on the population in electoral wards.

Jarman Index

The Jarman Index (1984) uses eight variables, weighted according to how much they are thought to reflect a population's need of general practice. The index was originally developed by asking general practitioners to list the contribution of census variables to their workload and it is used to determine extra deprivation payments for general practitioners. The variables are:

- Old people living alone
- Children aged under five years
- Single parent households
- Unskilled people
- Unemployed people
- Overcrowded households
- People who have moved house
- Ethnic minority households.

Townsend Score

The Townsend Score is used more frequently than the Jarman Index by public health workers and is also based on census data:

- % unemployed people
- % households with no car
- % households not owner-occupied
- % overcrowded households.

The practice age-sex register includes the patient's address and increasingly a postcode. This enables practice managers to evaluate their catchment population using the ACORN classification, and to compare this with other populations, such as the local district or Great Britain. ACORN is an acronym for A Classification Of Residential Neighbourhoods and is a composite socio-demographic index derived from census variables. Further information about ACORN is contained in the references at the end of this module. The advantage of this measure for general practice is that classification is available at enumeration level (about 300 persons) as compared to the Jarman and Townsend Indexes, which are only available to electoral ward level (about 8000 persons). The postcode in each patient's address identifies his/her enumeration district, and therefore the ACORN classification.

ACTIVITY DATA

Hospital information (including day cases and outpatients)

In England, the systems that are currently collecting hospital information are: (a) Hospital Management Information System (HMIS: Korner Aggregated Returns); and (b) Health Service Indicators (HSI).

Hospital Activity Analysis (HAA) became Korner Episode Statistics (KES) in 1987. HAA was a computerized system for recording all inpatient and day case activity other than maternity and psychiatry. Information can be obtained now from the Minimum Data Set (MDS) on length of consultant episode, age on admission, disposal on discharge, source and type of admission, and cases admitted from the waiting list. In addition, there is information on diagnosis (coded according to the International Classification of Diseases), type of operation (OPCS codes) and total length consultant episode (FCE). An MDS system for maternity is available.

The Hospital Management Information System (HMIS), now called the Korner Aggregated Returns System (KARS) is an administrative system. It records activity but does not record diagnoses or procedures carried out. VS forms are derived from this system. KARS data are usually recorded more completely than HAA.

The Mental Health Enquiry (MHE) system recorded information about the psychiatric patients discharged from hospital. It was replaced from April 1987 by a system similar to HAA.

The Scottish Morbidity Records, the SMR schemes, cover all outpatient attendances (SMR0), discharges from acute hospitals (SMR1), discharges from maternity units (SMR2), discharges from psychiatric wards (SMR4) and neonatal discharges (SMR11). SMR6 is a cancer register and SMR22/23 is the Scottish Drug Misuse Database. Tables are published annually in *Scottish Health Statistics* and an ad hoc enquiry service exists.

Hospital data also include waiting times. Monitoring the post-referral waiting time gives a more accurate figure than the waiting list data (Smith, 1994).

Data quality

Hospital data add to the health profile of a practice but may be problematic. In the past, the usefulness of hospital data has been limited by problems of incompleteness, inaccuracy and delays in publication (Kohli et al., 1992; Pearse et al., 1992; Denholm et al., 1993). There is renewed interest in the quality and timeliness of discharge data as they are utilized in the contracting process between provider units and fundholding general practices.

In addition, inpatient admission rates for most conditions are not a proxy for morbidity in the community. Payne et al. (1994b) examined the relationship between specific areas of morbidity measured using validated survey questionnaires (such as the MRC Respiratory Questionnaire) and hospital service usage. Only two diseases (respiratory disease and depression) out of the seven diseases or procedures investigated showed a positive correlation between hospital admission and disease prevalence rates. However, where two neighbourhoods are served by the same hospital, the relative bed usage may reflect comparative need.

Differences in hospital admission rates between districts, electoral wards or practice populations are thus the product of many factors:

- Most conditions are closely associated with variations in age, social class, and unemployment found in any population. This means that populations will differ both in their need and demand for health care and preventive services.

- Traditionally, areas with good access to hospital services in close proximity have higher admission rates than areas at greater distance.

- There are recognized variations in the practice of general practitioners referring to hospital and of hospital doctors accepting patients for admission.

- Some surgeons carry out procedures more readily than others, so that the number of operations carried out may reflect the practice of the surgeons rather than the need of the patients.

Nevertheless, admissions can be used as an initial step towards identifying need. Actual admissions for a range of surgical interventions in one practice's population can be compared with the rates for a district or region.

Child health computer systems

These provide community data in England. The Child Health Computer System was set up on a national basis; other systems have been adapted to meet local needs. They record details of every child aged 0–16 years old in a district. Births to local residents are recorded forming the mainstay of the system, supplemented by data from health visitors, general practitioners, schools, and school nurses, to maintain an accurate register of all resident children. The register is adjusted regularly for children who migrate in or out of the area and used to send appointments for immunizations and child health surveillance. Through this system, immunization uptake rates can be recorded.

Health Service Indicators

The Department of Health has been publishing a comparative information package since 1983 based on routine data submissions from throughout the NHS. The package compares performance indicators of provider units and health authorities, focusing attention on those falling in the outlier ranges (0–10%, 91%–100%). Highlighting extremes in this way helps providers to set targets. It also allows purchasers to compare the relative performance of providers.

The data are at least 18 months old and should be verified with more recent data before they influence decisions. Recent changes in the configuration of provider organizations may not be reflected in the package. Nevertheless, areas of high priority can easily be identified. Information on the DoH Performance Indicators can be obtained from the Department of Health, Room 1418, Euston Tower, 286 Euston Road, London NW1 3DN.

Health service activity in the community

General practitioners

Until recently little information was routinely collected on the activity of general practitioners. However, in the future, practice annual reports to the health authority should be a valuable source of information. In many districts, activity indicator packages are being developed along the lines of the IACC/Southampton Health Commission package described in Chapter 4 (page 20).

Community health services

Community health services include data on:

- Vaccination and immunization, obtainable from Korner statistics

- Family planning services, obtainable from Korner statistics

- School health services, obtainable from form 8MI

- Maternity and child health services, obtainable from Korner statistics.

HEALTH DATA

Health outcomes can be measured in a number of ways: for example, the mortality or morbidity resulting from a procedure, or the effect of a procedure on the quality of life. From the district point of view, mortality data are the easiest to obtain; death certificates of every resident who dies in the district, or elsewhere, are sent to the Director of Public Health. Morbidity data are more difficult to obtain. The decennial surveys of the Royal College of General Practitioners provide the most comprehensive data on morbidity in general practice.

Mortality data

Mortality in infancy

Statistics are subdivided as follows:

- Perinatal mortality rate—the number of stillbirths and deaths in the first week of life per 1000 total births

- Infant mortality rate—the number of deaths in the first year of life per 1000 live births.

As a generalization, perinatal mortality reflects the standards of health care provided to mother and infant; infant mortality reflects more the socio-economic conditions experienced in the first year of life. In recent years, nearly half of infant deaths have been attributed to sudden infant death syndrome (SIDS), or so-called 'cot deaths'. In 1992, the infant mortality rate for England and Wales fell to its lowest rate ever: 6.6 per 1000 live births (from 7.4 in 1991). This was due mainly to a 50% reduction in SIDS and a 40% reduction in deaths due to respiratory disease; this could mainly be attributed to the advice to put babies on their backs to sleep.

Standardized mortality ratios (SMRs)

A copy of the death certificate of everyone who dies is sent to the Director of Public Health. District mortality data contain some details of the number of people who died from a large number of conditions and are presented by age and sex, and place of death. Although the coverage of death certification in the UK is almost 100%, the quality of the information can be questioned. Comparison of the written death certificate with postmortem findings suggests that the clinical diagnosis can be incorrect.

To compare the mortality of local people with the rest of the population, data should be adjusted for age differences. A standardized mortality ratio expresses the number of deaths in a population as a ratio of those expected in that population if it had the same age-specific rates as the national population. Thus, an SMR of 120 means that the community has a mortality rate 20% above expected; an SMR of 80 is 20% below expected.

Standardized mortality ratios can be used as indicators of health at electoral ward level, or for comparisons of mortality from a specific cause. The measure becomes fairly meaningless if the number of deaths is small. Therefore its appropriateness for comparisons and trends depends on population size. At ward level, SMRs for all causes combined or the main causes of death such as coronary heart disease or neoplasm are therefore best aggregated, for example over three-year periods.

Morbidity data

Infectious disease

Episodes of notifiable infectious diseases are reported to the Local Authority Proper Officer, usually a consultant in communicable disease control. The Communicable Disease Surveillance Centre (CDSC) produces a weekly *Communicable Disease Report* (*CDR*) documenting the number of cases of notifiable infectious diseases which have been diagnosed in public health laboratories around the country.

There is evidence that infectious diseases are under-notified and there are some important infections that are not statutorily notifiable, for example HIV (which needs to be notified to OPCS).

Neoplastic disease

Incidence data on patients with malignant neoplasms and a few benign neoplasms are compiled by Cancer Registries. There are 14 of these in England and Wales.

Drug addiction

It is a legal requirement in England and Scotland to register with the Home Office every person known to be addicted to controlled drugs. This information is used to monitor the problem and to inform doctors if individuals are receiving treatment elsewhere.

Prescribable disease

Data on the number of prescribable (occupational certifiable) diseases are available from the Health and Safety Executive.

Incidence of disease in the community

There is no routine centralized system of measuring disease incidence in the community. Korner collects information on the diagnoses of people who are admitted to hospital, but in most conditions the number of hospital admissions for a condition is a poor measure of its incidence in the community. Not everyone with a given disease will be treated in hospital and Korner data reflect events rather than patients.

Conception rates

Conception rates comprise numbers of live births, stillbirths and terminations of pregnancy of particular age groups. There is no registration of miscarriages or spontaneous abortions. The rates are expressed as numbers per 1000 females in that age range. The most widely used are the age bands 11–15 years and 16–19 years as teenage pregnancies are thought to need more health care. One of the *Health of the Nation* targets is to reduce conception in girls under 16 by 50% by the year 2000. Fertility rates and total births are available by legitimacy, birthweight and social class from OPCS.

Various miscellaneous information sources primarily designed for purchasing authorities may occasionally be of interest at practice level. These include the Contract Minimum Data Set (CMDS), Developing Information Systems for Purchasers (DISP) and the Public Health Common Data Set for England and Wales. The latter draws together large quantities of demographic, fertility and mortality data pertaining to each health authority's resident population alongside aggregate regional and national figures. It highlights deaths from 'avoidable' and other potentially reducible causes of death. It includes statistics on population years of life lost attributable to selective causes of death. It is of particular value in comparing the health experience of your district with other parts of the country.

Interview schedule for residents

1. Community composition

- How long have you lived here?
- Do you know your neighbours?
- Do you have friends or relatives in this area that you see often?
- Can you describe the kinds of people who live in this area?
- Is the area better for some people to live in rather than others?

2. Socio-economic environment

- Are you aware of many people who find it hard to manage financially?
- How would you describe your own financial situation?
- Does your financial situation cause you any particular difficulties?
- How often do you get out . . . shopping . . . socializing?
- I'm sure you've heard reports on the TV and in the newspapers about domestic violence? Do you know if domestic violence is a problem in this area?

3. Community organization and structure

- Do you know what kind(s) of help is/are available for the residents of Dumbiedykes?
- Can you think of any other services which would be helpful to people in this area?

4. Community capacity

- Do you know of any local people who are good at getting things done?
- Do you think there is a sense of community identity and/or commitment to this area?
- Do you feel part of the community?

5. Physical environment

- Are there any particular problems with living in this area?
- How would you describe the condition of the housing in Dumbiedykes?
- Are there any particular problems with your house/flat?
- Does transport or access to the area present you with any problems?
- How safe do you feel in the neighbourhood, for example, walking outside after dark, or being at home alone; if not, why?
- Are you aware of any environmental health problems in the area?

6. Disease and disability profile

- What do you think are the worst health problems in the area?
- Have these changed over the last few years?
- Do you know if drug abuse is a problem?
- Do you know if alcohol abuse is a problem?
- Are there many people with a physical or learning disability living in the area?

7. Educational services

- Are you aware of these services available locally? (prompt list)
- How could they be improved?
- Is there anything else you would like in the area?

8. Health services

- Which of these medical services do you or have you used? (prompt list)
- What is the best thing about them and what could be better?
- Do you have any suggestions that would help to improve these services?
- What do you think of hospital services?
- Which hospital services do you use?
- Have you noticed any recent changes in these services?

9. Social services

- What social services do you use?
- What social services do people in the area use?
- What do you think of them?
- How would you like to see them improved?

10. Health policy

- There have been recent changes in the Health & Social Work Policy: have you received any of the following leaflets:
- *Patient's Charter?*
- *Community Care Plan?* (show leaflets)
- Have you read them?
- Do you think they will change anything?

11. Miscellaneous

- If you could wave a magic wand, what changes would you like to make in the area?
- Thinking about yourself and your family, has there ever been a time when you thought that help was not there when you needed it?
- Would you know where to get help?
- Is there anything you would like to ask or add?

References

Abramson JH (1988) Community-oriented primary care—strategy, approaches and practices. A review. *Public Health Review* **16**, 35–98.

Acheson D (1981) *Primary Health Care in Inner London*. London Health Planning Consortium. London, Department of Health and Social Security.

Acheson R (1988) *Public Health in England—the Report of the Committee of the Enquiry into the Future Development of the Public Health Function*. Cm 289. London, HMSO.

Annett H and Rifkin S (1995) Guidelines for rapid participatory appraisal to assess community health needs: a focus on health improvements for low income urban and rural areas. Geneva, World Health Organisation.

Ashton J (1990) Public health and primary care: towards a common agenda. *Public Health* **104**, 387–98.

Ashton J and Seymour H (1988) *The New Public Health*. Milton Keynes, Open University Press.

Audit Commission (1996) *What the Doctor Ordered. Fundholding: The Main Report*. London, HMSO.

Baker D and Klein R (1991) Explaining outputs of primary health care: population and practice factors. *British Medical Journal* **303**, 225–9.

Berlin A, Bhopal R, Spencer J et al. (1993) Creating a death register for general practice. *British Journal of General Practice* **43**, 70–72.

Bero LA, Galbraith A and Rennie D (1992) The publication of sponsored symposiums in medical journals. *New England Journal of Medicine* **327**, 1135-40.

Berridge V (1991) *A History of Public Health*. London, Oxford University Press. Ch. 3.

Bhopal R (1995) Public health medicine and primary health care: convergent, divergent or parallel? *Journal of Epidemiology and Community Health* **49**, 113–6.

Black D, Birchall A and Trimble I (1994) Non-fundholding in Nottingham: a vision of the future. *British Medical Journal* **309**, 930–2.

Black N (1996) Why we need observational studies to evaluate the effectiveness of health care. *British Medical Journal* **312**, 1215–8.

Blaxter M (1995) Consumer issues within the NHS. Leeds, NHSE Research & Development Directorate.

Bowling A (1991) *Measuring Health. A Review of Quality of Life Measurement Scales*. Milton Keynes, Open University Press.

Bowling A (1996) Health care rationing: the public's debate. *British Medical Journal* **312**, 670–4.

Bowling A, Jacobsen B and Southgate L (1993) Health Services priorities. Exploration in consultation of the public and health professionals on priority setting in an inner London health district. *Social Science and Medicine* **37**, 851–7.

Boyle P, Muir CS and Grundman E (1989) Cancer mapping. *Recent Results in Cancer Research* **114**.

Boyle S (1993) Ghostbusters. *Health Service Journal* **103**, 24–25.

Bradshaw JS (1972) A taxonomy of social need. In McLachlan G (Ed.). *Problems and Progress in Medical Care: Essays on Current Research*. 7th series. London, Oxford University Press.

Brazier JE, Harper R, Jones NMB et al. (1992) Validating the SF-36 health survey questionnaire: new outcome measure for primary care. *British Medical Journal* **305**, 160–4.

Britten N and Fisher B (1993) Qualitative research and general practice. *British Journal of General Practice* **43**, 270–1.

Brody H (1992) Philosophic approaches. In Crabtree B and Miller W (Eds). *Doing Qualitative Research: Multiple Strategies*. London, Sage Publications. Ch. 9.

Butler J (1989) *Child Health Surveillance in Primary Care*. London, HMSO.

Carlisle RD, Jonstone SP and Pearson JCG (1993) Relation between night visit rates and deprivation measures in one general practice. *British Medical Journal* **306**, 1383–5.

Cartwright A (1986) Some experiments with factors that might affect the response of mothers to a postal questionnaire. *Statistics in Medicine* **5**, 607–17.

Chambers R (1983) *Rural Development: Putting the Last First*. London, Longman.

Charlton BG, Calvert N and White M (1994) Health promotion priorities for general practice; constructing and using "indicative prevalences". *British Medical Journal* **308**, 1019–22.

Chisholm J (1990) The Read Clinical Classification: The NHS has acquired a coding system designed for the computer age. *British Medical Journal* **300**, 1092–4.

Colledge M and Morse D (1995) *Strategic Planning in General Practice: Mapping the Health Care Needs of a Community*. Department of General Practice, University of Glasgow.

Coulter A (1992) Fundholding general practices: early successes but will they last? *British Medical Journal* **304**, 397–8.

Coulter A (1995) Evaluating general practitioner fundholding. *European Journal of Public Health* **5**, 233–9.

Crabtree BF and Miller WL (1992) *Doing Qualitative Research: Multiple Strategies. Research Methods for Primary Care*. **Vol. 3**. London, Sage Publications.

Cresswell T (1992) Assessing community health and social needs in North Derbyshire using participatory rapid appraisal. *Medical Sociology News* **17**, 27–38.

Culyer AJ (1976) *Need and the National Health Service*. London, Martin Robertson.

Currer C (1991) The case of pathan women in Britain, in child health matters. In Wyke S and Hewison J (Eds). *Understanding the Mother's Viewpoint*. Milton Keynes, Open University Press.

Davey Smith G (1991) Second thoughts on the Jarman Index. *British Medical Journal* **302**, 359–60.

Day P (1992) The State, the NHS and general practice. *Journal of Public Health Policy* **13**, 165–79.

Day P and Klein R (1991) Variations in budgets of fundholding practices. *British Medical Journal* **303**, 168–70.

Denholm SW, Macintyre CCA and Wilson JA (1993) Audit of the Scottish Morbidity Record 1 (SMR1). Returns from an ENT Unit. *Health Bulletin* **51**, 366–9.

Department of Health (1992) *The Health of the Nation: A Strategy for Health in England*. London, HMSO.

Department of Health (1993a) *Research for Health*. London, Department of Health.

Department of Health (1993b) *Population Health Outcome Indicators for the NHS, England—a Consultation Document*. London, Department of Health.

Department of Health (1993c) *Public Health Commission Data Set*. 14 regional volumes. London, Department of Health.

Department of Health, Department of Social Security, Welsh Office and Scottish Office (1990) *Caring for People*. London, HMSO.

Department of Health and the Welsh Office (1989) *General Practice in the National Health Service: A New Contract*. London, HMSO.

Dixon J (1994) Can there be fair funding for fundholding practices? *British Medical Journal* **308**, 772–5.

Dixon J, Dinwoodie M, Hodson D et al. (1994) Distribution of NHS funds between fundholding and non-fundholding practices. *British Medical Journal* **309**, 30-34.

Dixon J and Glennerster H (1995) What do we know about fundholding in general practice? *British Medical Journal* **311**, 727–30.

Drummond MF (1980) *Principles of Economic Appraisal in Health Care.* Oxford, Oxford University Press.

Eddy D (1991) Where is the wisdom . . .? The poverty of medical evidence. *British Medical Journal* **303**, 798-9.

Field K, Thorogood M, Silagy C et al. (1995) Strategies for coronary risk factor prevention in primary care: which is the most cost-effective? *British Medical Journal* **310**, 1109–12.

Fitzpatrick R, Fletcher A, Gore S et al. (1992) Quality of life measures in health care. I: Applications and issues in assessment. *British Medical Journal* **305**, 1074–7.

Fowler G and Mant D (1990) Health checks for adults. *British Medical Journal* **300**, 1318–20.

Frankel SJ (1992) Health needs, health care requirements, and the myth of infinite demand. *Lancet* **337**, 1588–9.

Fry J (1993) *General Practice. The Facts.* Oxford, Radcliffe Medical Press.

Fullard E, Fowler G and Gray JAM (1987) Promoting prevention in primary care. A controlled trial of a low technology, low cost approach. *British Medical Journal* **194**, 1080–2.

Garratt AM, Ruta DA, Abdalla MI et al. (1993) The SF 36 health survey questionnaire: an outcome measure suitable for routine use within the NHS. *British Medical Journal* **306**, 1440–4.

Geiger HJ (1983) The meaning of community-oriented primary care in an American context. In Connor E and Mullan F (Eds). *Community-oriented Primary Care: New Directions for Health Services Delivery: Conference Proceedings.* Washington DC, National Academy Press.

General Medical Council (1993) *Tomorrow's Doctors. Recommendations on Undergraduate Medical Education.* London, GMC.

General Medical Services Committee and RCGP Joint Computing Group (1988) *The Classification of General Practice Data.* Final report of the GMSC-RCGP Joint Computing Group Technical Working Party. London, GMSC, BMA.

Gill P, Dowell A, Neal R et al. (1996) Evidence-based general practice: a retrospective study of interventions in one training practice. *British Medical Journal* **312**, 819–21.

Gill TM (1994) Quality-of-life measurements miss the mark. *Journal of the American Medical Association* **272**, 619–26.

Gillam SJ (1992a) Provision of health promotion clinics in relation to population need: another example of the inverse care law? *British Journal of General Practice* **42**, 54–56.

Gillam SJ (1992b) Assessing populations' health needs: the general practitioner's contribution. *British Journal of General Practice* **42**, 404–5.

Gillam SJ, Plamping D, McClenahan J et al. (1994) *Community-oriented Primary Care.* London, King's Fund.

Glennerster H, Matsaganis M and Owens P (1994) *Implementing GP Fundholding: Wild Card or Winning Hand?* Buckingham, Open University Press.

Gooding S (1991) Community Participation in General Practice. MSc thesis. London, King's College.

Graffy J and Williams J (1994) Purchasing for all: an alternative to fundholding. *British Medical Journal* **308**, 391–4.

Gray DP, Steele R, Sweeney K et al. (1994) Generalists in medicine. *British Medical Journal* **308**, 486–7.

Grimshaw JM and Russell IT (1993) Effect of clinical guidelines on medical practice: a systematic review of rigorous evaluations. *Lancet* **342**, 1317–22.

Gudex C (1986) *QALYs and their Use by the Health Service. Discussion Paper 20.* York, Centre for Health Economics.

Haines A and Jones R (1994) Implementing findings of research. *British Medical Journal* **308**, 1488–92.

Hall DB (Ed.) (1992) *Health For All Children.* Joint Working Party on Child Health Surveillance. Oxford, Oxford University Press.

Ham C (1993) *Locality Purchasing. Discussion Paper 34.* Institute of Health Services Management, University of Birmingham.

Ham C and Shapiro J (1995) The future of fundholding. *British Medical Journal* **310**, 1150–1.

Handysides S (1994) New roles for general practitioners. *British Medical Journal* **308**, 513–6.

Hanlon A and Hargreaves S (1994) Performance indicators for general practice. *Journal of Epidemiology and Community Health* **48**, 502.

Hannay DR (1993) Primary care and public health: too far apart. *British Medical Journal* **307**, 516–7.

Hart JT (1988) *A New Kind of Doctor.* London, Merlin Press.

Hart JT (1990a) Coronary heart disease prevention in primary care: seven lessons from three decades. *Family Practice* **7**, 288–94.

Hart JT (1990b) Reactive and proactive care: a crisis. James Mackenzie Lecture 1989. *Journal of the Royal College of General Practitioners* **40**, 4–10.

Hart JT, Thomas C, Gibbons B et al. (1991) Twenty five years of case funding and audit in a socially deprived community. *British Medical Journal* **302**, 1509–13.

Health Promotion Research Trust (1993) *The Health and Lifestyle Survey; Seven years on: a Review.* Cambridge, Health Promotion Trust.

Helman C (1984) *Culture, Health and Illness.* Bristol, Wright.

Heritage Z (Ed.) (1994) *Community Participation in Primary Care. Occasional Paper 64.* London, Royal College of General Practitioners.

Honigsbaum F, Callthorp J, Ham C et al. (1995) *Priority Setting for Health Care.* Oxford, Radcliffe Medical Press.

Hopton JL and Dlugolecka M (1995) Patients' perceptions of need for primary health care services: useful for priority setting? *British Medical Journal* **310**, 1237–40.

Hopton JL, Howie JGR and Porter M (1992) Social indicators of health needs for general practice: a simpler approach. *British Journal of General Practice* **42**, 236–40.

Hopton JL, Porter M and Howie JGR (1991) A measure of perceived health in evaluating general practice: the Nottingham Health Profile. *Family Practice* **8**, 253–9.

Howie JGR, Heaney DJ and Maxwell M (1994) Evaluating care of patients reporting pain in fundholding practices. *British Medical Journal* **309**, 705–10.

Howie JGR, Heaney D and Maxwell M (1995) Care of patients with selected health problems in fundholding practices in Scotland in 1990 and 1992: needs, process and outcome. *British Journal of General Practice* **45**, 121–6.

Hsiao W, Braun P, Dunn D et al. (1988) Results and policy implications of the resource-based relative value study. *New England Journal of Medicine* **319**, 881–8.

Hume D (1995) *Deprivation in Lothian Region: An Analysis of 1991 Census Data.* Edinburgh, Lothian Regional Council.

Hunt SM, McEwen J and McKenna SP (1985) Social inequalities and perceived health. *Effective Health Care* **2**, 151–9.

Hunt SM, McEwen J and McKenna SP (1986) *Measuring Health Status.* London, Croom Helm.

Hunter D (1994) Are we being effective? *Health Service Journal,* 16 June, p. 23.

Illich I (1975) *Medical Nemesis—the Expropriation of Health.* London, Marion Boyars.

Imperial Cancer Research Fund OXCHECK Study Group (1995) Effectiveness of health checks conducted by nurses in primary care: final results of the OXCHECK study. *British Medical Journal* **310**, 1099–1104.

Jarman B (1984) Underprivileged areas: validation and distribution of scores. *British Medical Journal* **229**, 1587–92.

Johnson JC (1990) *Selecting Ethnographic Informants*. London, Sage Publications.

Jones R (1995) Why do qualitative research? It should begin to close the gap between the sciences of discovery and implementation. *British Medical Journal* **311**, 2

Kark SL (1981) *The Practices of Community Orientated Primary Health Care*. New York, Appleton-Century-Crofts.

Kennedy A (1994) Practising Health for All in a Glasgow Housing Scheme. Glasgow, Drumchapel Community Health Project.

Kickbusch I (1986) Health promotion strategies for action. *Canadian Journal of Public Health* **77**, 321–6.

Kingdom D and Sumners S (1995) Community care and general practice. *British Medical Journal* **311**, 823–4.

Kohli HS and Knill-Jones RP (1992) How accurate are SMR1 (Scottish Morbidity Record 1) data? *Health Bulletin* **50**, 14–23.

Lalonde M (1974) *The New Perspective on the Health of Canadians*. Canada, Ministry of Supply and Services.

Langham S, Thorogood M, Normand C et al. (1996) Costs and cost effectiveness of health checks conducted by nurses in primary care: the OXCHECK study. *British Medical Journal* **312**, 1265–8.

Last JM (1963) The iceberg: completing the clinical picture in general practice. *Lancet* **2**, 28–31.

Le Grand J (1994) Evaluating the NHS reforms. In Robinson R and Le Grand J (Eds). *Evaluating the NHS Reforms*. London, King's Fund Institute.

McCormick A, Charlton J and Fleming D (1995) Assessing health needs in primary care: Morbidity study from general practice provides another source of information. *British Medical Journal* **310**, 1534.

McKeown T (1976) *The Role of Medicine—Dream, Mirage, Nemesis*. London, Nuffield Provincial Hospitals Trust.

Majeed FA and Voss S (1995) Performance indicators for general practice. *British Medical Journal* **311**, 209–10.

Mant D and Anderson P (1985) Community general practitioner. *Lancet* **2**, 1114–7.

Marinker M (1967) Studies of contact in a general practice. *Journal of the Royal College of General Practitioners* **14**, 59.

Marsh GN and Channing DM (1988) Narrowing the health gap between a deprived and an endowed community. *British Medical Journal* **296**, 173–6.

Matthew GK (1972) Measuring need and evaluating services. In McLachlan G (Ed.). *Portfolio for Health*. Oxford, Oxford University Press.

Metcalfe DH (1990) Measurement of outcomes in general practice. In Hopkins A and Costain D. *Measuring the Outcomes of Medical Care*. London, Royal College of Physicians/King's Fund Centre for Health Services Development.

Milne R (1995) Developing critical appraisal skills. *Health Services Journal*, 24 April, pp 24–25.

Mooney GH (1986) *Economics, Medicine and Health Care*. Brighton, Harvest Press.

Mulrow CD (1987) The medical review article: state of the science. *Annals of Internal Medicine* **106**, 485–8.

Murphy E and Mattson B (1992) Qualitative research and family practice: a marriage made in heaven? *Family Practice* **9**, 85–91.

Murray E and Modell M (1995) General practice: the ideal place to teach general medicine? Student perceptions of a community based junior medical firm. *Family Practice* **12**, 266.

Murray S (1995) A critical assessment of the use of rapid participatory appraisal to assess health needs in a small neighbourhood. MD thesis. University of Aberdeen.

Murray S and Graham L (1995) Practice based health needs assessment: use of four methods in a small neighbourhood. *British Medical Journal* **310**, 1443–8.

Murray S, Graham L and Dlugolecka M (1995) How many general practitioners for 1433 patients? *British Medical Journal* **310,** 1443–8.

Neve H and Taylor P (1995) Working with the community. *British Medical Journal* **311**, 524–5.

Newton J, Fraser M, Robinson J et al. (1993) Fundholding in Northern region: the first year. *British Medical Journal* **306,** 375–8.

NHS Centre for Coding and Classification (1993) *Read Codes and the Terms Projects: a Brief Guide*. London, Department of Health.

NHS Management Executive (1991) *Assessing Health Care Needs*. A DHA Project Discussion Paper, EL(91)41, May.

NHS Management Executive (1992) *Local Voices*. The views of local people in purchasing for health. London, NHSME.

NHS Management Executive (1993a) *Improving Clinical Effectiveness*. EL(93)115. Leeds, NHSME.

NHS Management Executive (1993b) GP contract health promotion package: an amendment to the statement of fees and allowances. FHSL(93)25. London, Department of Health.

NHS Executive (1994) *Developing NHS Purchasing and GP Fundholding*. EL(94)79. London, Department of Health.

NHS Executive (1995) *Improving the Effectiveness of Clinical Services*. EL(95)105. Leeds, NHSE.

NHS Management Executive (1995) *Assessing the Options: CHD/Stroke. Target—Effectiveness of Interventions to Reduce CHD and Stroke Mortality*. London, Department of Health.

NHS Training Division (1994) Health needs assessment and health gain. In Anonymous (Ed.) *Rainbow III: Using Information in Practice Management*. Yorkshire, Greenhalgh.

Nutting P (1987) *Community-Oriented Primary Care: From Principles to Practice*. Albuquerque, University of New Mexico Press.

Oakley P (1989) *Community Involvement in Health Development, An Examination of the Critical Issues*. Geneva, World Health Organisation.

Old P, Voss S and Davidge M (1994) Performing arts. *Health Service Journal* **104**, 288–9.

Ong BN, Humphris G, Annett H et al. (1992) Rapid appraisal in an urban setting, an example from the developed world. *Social Science and Medicine* **32**, 909–15.

Office of Population Censuses and Surveys (1993) *General Household Survey 1989*. London, HMSO.

Office of Population Censuses and Surveys (1992) *Census 1991—Key Statistics for Local Authorities*. London, HMSO.

Open University (1991) Managing health services. Book 9. In *Managing Change*. Milton Keynes, Open Business School.

Oswald NT (1989) Why not base medical education in general practice? *Lancet* **2**, 148–9.

Oxman AD, Sackett D and Guyatt G (1994) Users' guides to the medical literature. *Journal of the American Medical Association* **270**, 2093–5.

Payne N, Jones G, Norris J et al. (1994a) Profiling general practices. *British Journal of Health Care Computing and Information Management* **11**, 12–13.

Payne JN, Coy J, Patterson S et al. (1994b) Is use of hospital services a proxy for morbidity? A small area comparison of the prevalence of arthritis, depression, dyspepsia, obesity, and respiratory disease with inpatient admission rates for these disorders in England. *Journal of Epidemiology and Community Health* **48**, 74–78.

Pearse J, Alexander V, Alexander GF et al. (1992) Audit of the quality of hospital discharge data. *Health Bulletin* **50**, 356–61.

Pearson P, O'Brien J, Thomas H et al. (1996) Collecting morbidity data in general practice: the Somerset morbidity project. *British Medical Journal* **312**, 1517–20.

Plant R (1987) *Managing Change and Making it Stick*. London, Fontana.

Pope C and Mays N (1995) Reaching the parts other methods cannot reach: an introduction to qualitative methods in health and health services research. *British Medical Journal* **311**, 42–46.

Pringle M and Hobbs R (1991) Large computer databases in general practice. *British Medical Journal* **302**, 741–2.

Pringle M, Bilkhu JAS, Dornan M et al. (1991) *Managing Change in General Practice*. Oxford, Radcliffe Medical Press.

Pritchard P (1981) *Patient Participation in General Practice. Occasional Paper 17*. London, Royal College of General Practitioners.

Pritchard P (1993) *Partnership with Patients*. London, Royal College of General Practitioners.

Record M, Spencer JA, Jones RH et al. (1994) General practitioners' views about the statutory annual practice report. *British Medical Journal* **309**, 849–52.

Reid DA (1992) GPs' recognition of need in the community. Letter. *British Journal of General Practice* **42**, 258–9.

Rennie D and Bero LA (1990) Throw it away, Sam: the controlled circulation journals. *CBE Views* **13**, 31–35.

Rifkin SSB (1992) Rapid appraisals for health: a overview. In Welbourne I (Ed.) *RRA Notes. No 16: Special Issue on Applications for Health*. London, International Institution for Environment and Development.

Rogers D (1982) Community-oriented primary care. *Journal of the American Medical Association* **248**, 1622–5.

Robson J, Falshaw M and Healthy Eastenders Project (1995) Audit of preventive activities in 16 inner London practices using a validated measure of patient population, the active patient denominator. *British Journal of General Practice* **45**, 463–6.

Roland M and Coulter A (Eds) (1993) *Hospital Referrals*. Oxford, Oxford University Press.

Rose G (1992) *The Strategy of Preventive Medicine*. Oxford, Oxford University Press.

Royal College of General Practitioners (1995) *Fellowship By Assessment. Occasional Paper 50*. 2nd edn. London, RCGP.

Royal College of Nursing (1993) *The GP Practice Population Profile*. A framework for every member of the primary health care team. London, RCN.

Russell EM (1988) Community medicine and primary care in Scotland. *Community Medicine* **10**, 112–6.

Saunders D, Coulter A and McPherson K (1989) *Variation in Hospital Admission Rates, A Review of the Literature*. London, King's Fund Centre.

Schofield T (1992) Health promotion in primary care—does teamwork make a difference? *Journal of Interprofessional Care* **6**, 97–101.

Secretary of State for Health (1989) *Working for Patients*. Cm 555. London, HMSO.

Secretary of State for Social Services (1987) *Promoting Better Health*. Cm 249. London, HMSO.

Shanks J, Kheraj S and Fish S (1995) Better way of assessing health needs in primary care. *British Medical Journal* **310**, 480–1.

Shapiro J (1994) *Shared Purchasing and Collaborative Commissioning within the NHS*. Birmingham, National Association of Health Authorities and Trusts.

Sheikh K and Mattingly S (1981) Investigating nonresponse bias in mail surveys. *Journal of Epidemiology and Community Health* **35**, 293–6.

Sheldon T, Seith P, Borowitz M et al. (1994) Attempt at deriving a formula for setting general practitioner fundholding budgets. *British Medical Journal* **309**, 1059–64.

Smith N, Wilson A and Weekes T (1995) Use of Read codes in development of a standard database. *British Medical Journal* **311**, 313–5.

Smith T (1994) Waiting times; monitoring the total post-referral wait. *British Medical Journal* **309**, 593–6.

Smith WCS (1985) Comparison of response rates to a postal questionnaire from a general practice and research unit. *British Medical Journal* **291**, 1483–5.

Smith WCS, Lee AJ, Crombie JK et al. (1990) Control of blood pressure in Scotland: the rule of halves. *British Medical Journal* **300**, 8981–3.

Spiegel N, Murphy E, Kinmonth AL et al. (1992) Managing change in general practice: a step by step guide. *British Medical Journal* **304**, 231–4.

Stevens A and Gabbay J (1991) Needs assessment, needs assessment . . . *Health Trends* **23**, 20–23.

Stevens A and Raftery J (1993) *Health Care Needs Assessment—The Epidemiologically Based Needs Assessment Reviews*. Oxford, Radcliffe Medical Press.

Stott NCH and Pill R (1990) 'Advice Yes, Dictate No': patients' views on health promotion in the consultation. *Family Practice* **17**, 125–31.

Sykes W, Collins M, Hunter D et al. (1992) *Listening to Local Voices: A Guide to Research Methods*. Leeds, NHS Management Executive.

Taylor M, Milne B, Glen J et al. (1993) GPASS Data Evaluation Project Aberdeen. Unpublished.

Taylor R (1996) Experts and evidence. *British Journal of General Practice* **46**, 268-70.

Toon P (1994) *What is Good General Practice? Occasional Paper 65*. London, Royal College of General Practitioners.

Twinn S, Dauncey J and Carnell J (1992) *The Process of Health Profiling*. London, Health Visitors' Association.

Wagstaff R, Berlin A, Stacy R et al. (1994) Information about patients' deaths: general practitioners' current practice and views on receiving death register. *British Journal of General Practice* **44**, 315–6.

Walsh K (1994) Evaluation of the use of general practice age-sex registers in epidemiological research. *British Journal of General Practice* **44**, 118–22.

Wearne M (1993) The Role of the Public Health Nurse in Needs Assessment. Castlefields Health Centre. MSc Dissertation.

Wennberg JE, Malley AG, Hanley D et al. (1988) An assessment of prostatectomy for benign urinary tract obstruction. Geographic variations and the evaluation of medical care outcomes. *Journal of the American Medical Association* **259**, 3027–30.

White KL (1976) Primary care research and the new epidemiology. Editorial. *Journal of Family Practice* **3**, 579–80.

White KL, Williams TF and Greenberg BG (1961) The ecology of medical care. *New England Journal of Medicine* **265**, 885–92.

Whitty P and Jones I (1992) Public health heresy: a challenge to the purchasing orthodoxy. *British Medical Journal* **304**, 1039–41.

Wilkin D, Hallam L and Doggett M (1992) *Measures of Need and Outcome in Primary Health Care*. London, Oxford Medical Publication.

Williams A (1976) Need—an economic exegesis. In Culyer AJ and Wright KG (Eds). *Economic Aspects of Health Services*. London, Martin Robertson.

Williams A (1989) *Creating a Health Care Market; Ideology, Efficacy, Ethics and Clinical Freedom*. York, Centre for Health Economics, University of York.

Wilson A (1995) *Final Report of the Wakefield and Pontefract Primary Care Health Information Project (WAPPCHIP)*. University of Leeds, Centre for Research in Primary Care.

Wilson AE, Pollock C, Weekes T et al. (1995) Can general practice provide useful information? Evaluation of a primary health care information project in northern England. *Journal of Epidemiology and Community Health* **49**, 227–30.

Wonderling D, McDermott C, Buxton M et al. (1996) Costs and cost effectiveness of cardiovascular screening and intervention: the British Family Heart Study. *British Medical Journal* **312**, 1269–73.

Wood DA, Kinmonth AL, Pyke SD et al. (1994) A randomised controlled trial evaluating cardiovascular screening and intervention in general practice: principal results of the British Family Heart Study. *British Medical Journal* **308**, 313–20.

World Health Organisation (1978) *Primary Health Care.* A joint report by the Director-General of the World Health Organisation and the Executive Director of the United Nations Children's Fund. Geneva, WHO.

World Health Organisation (1981) *Global Strategy for Health for All by the Year 2000.* Geneva, WHO.

Wright R (1993) Community-oriented primary care. The cornerstone of health care reform. *Journal of the American Medical Association* **269**, 2544–7.

Glossary

Bias is the deviation of results from the truth, due to systematic error(s) in the methods used.

Clinical effectiveness is the extent to which a treatment, procedure or service does patients more good than harm. Ideally, the determination of clinical effectiveness is based on the results of a randomized controlled trial. This is also known simply as '**effectiveness**'.

Cochrane Collaboration is an endeavour in which people from many different countries systematically find, appraise and review available evidence from randomized controlled trials. The Cochrane Collaboration's aims are to develop and maintain systematic, up-to-date reviews of randomized controlled trials of all forms of health care and to make this information readily available to clinicians and other decision-makers at all levels of health care systems. Areas which have been reviewed to date include effective care in pregnancy and childbirth, and stroke. The UK Cochrane Centre is based in Summertown in Oxford.

Confidence interval is the range within which the true size of effect (never exactly known) lies with a given degree of assurance. People often speak of a "95% confidence interval" (or "95% confidence limits"). This is the interval which includes the true value in 95% of cases.

Controls in a randomized controlled trial are people in a comparison group. They are allocated a different treatment from the subjects of the study.

Critical appraisal is the process of assessing and interpreting evidence by systematically considering its validity, results and relevance to one's own work.

Homogeneity means 'similarity'. Studies are said to be homogeneous if their results vary no more than might be expected by the play of chance. The opposite of homogeneity is **heterogeneity.**

Locality planning refers to the process of bringing general practitioners and others together from clusters of practices in the same geographical locality to provide advice to health authority planners. Different models exist. Locality purchasing (or commissioning) extends this process to include responsibility for a budget and may provide an alternative to fundholding.

MEDLINE is an electronic database which summarizes thousands of pieces of biomedical research literature published in selected journals. It is available through most health service libraries. It can be accessed by CD-ROM, through 'Datastar', by telephone and by other means.

Meta-analysis is a statistical technique which summarizes the results of several studies into a single estimate, giving more weight to results from larger studies.

Number needed to treat is one measure of a treatment's clinical effectiveness. It is the number of people that need to be treated with a specific intervention (for example, aspirin for people having a heart attack) to see one occurrence of a specific outcome (for example, prevention of death).

Odds ratio is one measure of a treatment's clinical effectiveness. If it is equal to 1, then the effects of the treatment are no different from those of the control treatment. If the odds ratio is greater (or less) than 1, then the effects of the treatment are more (or less) then those of the control treatment. It should be noted that the effects being measured may be adverse (for example, death, disability) or desirable (for example, stopping smoking).

Publication bias results from the fact that studies with 'positive' results are more likely to be published.

A randomized controlled trial is a trial in which subjects are randomly assigned to two groups: one (the experimental group) receiving the intervention that is being tested, and the other (the comparison group or controls) receiving an alternative treatment. The two groups are then followed up to see if any differences between them result. This helps people to assess the effectiveness of the intervention.

A review is any summary of the literature.

A systematic review is a review in which evidence on a topic has been systematically identified, appraised and summarized according to predetermined criteria. (Some people call this an 'overview'.)

Validity refers to the soundness or rigour of a study. A study is valid if the way it is designed and carried out means that the results are unbiased—that is, it gives a 'true' estimate of clinical effectiveness.

COLLEGE PUBLICATIONS

Medicine and Society

Alcohol — A Balanced View (Report 24)
A logical approach to drinking problems which can easily be applied in everyday practice. £5.00 (£5.50 non-members)

Patients and their Doctors 1977 (Occasional Paper 8)
Cartwright and Anderson follow up their classic work on patients' views of their doctors. £3.00 (£3.30 non-members)

A Survey of Primary Care in London (Occasional Paper 16)
Detailed documentation on the illness and social conditions of patients in London and the characteristics of their GPs and other health services. £4.00 (£4.40 non-members)

Inner Cities (Occasional Paper 19)
Prize-winning report, analysing the problems of general practice in several inner cities. £3.00 (£3.30 non-members)

General Practitioner Hospitals (Occasional Paper 23)
A working party reviews the history and literature on GP hospitals. £3.00 (£3.30 non-members)

Social Class and Health Status: Inequality or Difference (Occasional Paper 25)
Evidence that GPs provide more care for patients in social classes 4 and 5. £3.50 (£3.85 non-members)

Booking for Maternity Care. A Comparison of Two Systems (Occasional Paper 31)
A detailed study of the views of mothers booked for delivery in a GP unit and those booked for shared care in a specialist consultant unit. £3.50 (£3.85 non-members)

Community Hospitals (Occasional Paper 43)
An essential text for those involved in community hospitals who wish to learn more about them. A companion to Occasional Paper 23. £8.50 (£9.35 non-members)

Report of the Inner City Task Force of the RCGP (Occasional Paper 66)
Reports the results of a survey, identifies problems and makes recommendations for action. £10.00 (£11.00 non-members)

To Heal or to Harm
Describes the theory of somatic fixation and how doctors, patients, and others contribute to this; also practical ways in which it can be prevented. £12.50 (£13.75 non-members)

Forty Years On–the Story of the First Forty Years of the RCGP
This large, well-illustrated book traces the achievements of the College from its inception. £18.00 (£20.00 non-members)

Partnership with Patients
This 3rd edition offers practical guidance on starting a patient participation group and evaluates the achievements of patient participation. £6.00 (£6.60 non-members)

Rural General Practice in the UK (Occasional Paper 71)
An overview of the problems and potential of rural practice. £10.00 (£11.50 non-members)

All the above can be obtained from the Sales Office, Royal College of General Practitioners, 14 Princes Gate, London SW7 1PU. Prices include postage. Cheques should be made payable to the Royal College of General Practitioners. Access and Visa are welcome (Tel: 0171-225 3048).

COLLEGE PUBLICATIONS

Teamwork

Prevention and the Primary Care Team
A multidisciplinary working party looks at some of the difficulties in prevention and makes practical recommendations. £3.00 (£3.30 non-members)

Healthier Children — Thinking Prevention (Report 22)
Covers many principles involved in child care: examinations, doctor-patient relationship, teamwork, remuneration, monitoring and training. £5.50 (£6.05 non-members)

Education for Co-operation in Health and Social Work (Occasional Paper 14)
Reports an interdisciplinary conference of social workers, nurses, health visitors and GPs: how they can co-operate and the difficulties involved. £3.00 (£3.30 non-members)

Promoting Prevention (Occasional Paper 22)
Practical ways of carrying out prevention through teamwork in the practice and partnership with other health service organizations. £3.00 (£3.30 non-members)

Working Together — Learning Together (Occasional Paper 33)
Reports successes and failures of courses run to promote teamwork in general practice. £3.00 (£3.30 non-members)

Preventive Care of the Elderly (Occasional Paper 35)
Based on a national workshop, this document describes case-finding and screening programmes for the elderly, with special emphasis on team care. £5.00 (£5.50 non-members)

Care of Old People: A Framework for Progress (Occasional Paper 45)
A College working party describes challenges in caring for the elderly in relation to the new contract and makes recommendations for good practice. £7.00 (£7.70 non-members)

Primary Care for People with a Mental Handicap (Occasional Paper 47)
A College working party with multiprofessional authorship tackles the problems facing people with mental handicap, making important recommendations about improving their care. £7.50 (£8.25 non-members)

Shared Care of Patients with Mental Health Problems (Occasional Paper 60)
The report of a joint working party of the RCGP and Royal College of Psychiatrists. £6.00 (£6.60 non-members)

Community Participation in Primary Care (Occasional Paper 64)
A multidisciplinary paper from the HEA Primary Health Care Unit at Oxford describing the principles and practice of community participation. £9.00 (£9.90 non-members)

Shared Care for Diabetes (Occasional Paper 67)
A systematic review of 22 schemes sharing care between GPs and specialists. £9.00 (£9.90 non-members)

All the above can be obtained from the Sales Office, Royal College of General Practitioners, 14 Princes Gate, London SW7 1PU. Prices include postage. Cheques should be made payable to the Royal College of General Practitioners. Access and Visa are welcome (Tel: 0171-225 3048).

Education for General Practice

Editor
Declan Dwyer
167 North Road West, Plymouth PL1 5BZ, UK

Assistant Editor
Paul Sackin, *Huntingdon*

Editorial Board
Jamie Bahrami, *Leeds*. John Bligh, *Liverpool*.
Graham Buckley, *Edinburgh*. Peter Burrows,
Southampton. Peter Campion, *Liverpool*. Peter
Havelock, *High Wycombe*. Lesley Millard,
Southampton. Roger Neighbour, *Watford*. Janet
Perks, *Plymouth*. William Reith, *Aberdeen*. John
Salinsky, *London*. Paul Wright, *Dorchester*.

Overseas Editorial Board
John Frey, *Wisconsin, USA*. Richard Hays, *Queensland, Australia*. Tom O'Dowd,
Dublin, Ireland. Jack Rodnick, *San Fransisco, USA*. Chris van Weel, *Nijmegen,
The Netherlands*.

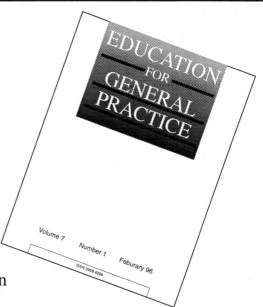

Volume 7   Number 1   Feburary 96

ISSN 0959 4299

Education for General Practice is the professional journal for all those involved
in GP education including undergraduate and vocational training and continuing
medical education. It has a substantial, fully-paid subscription which enjoys steady
growth in both the UK and overseas. The journal aims:

- to publish articles on medical educational
  method, content and assessment

- to provide information on teaching
  methods and content to those organizing
  courses for the continuing education of
  established general practitioners

- to promote a link between training
  practices and vocational training schemes

- to improve the one-to-one teaching skills
  of general practitioner trainers

- to provide an academic forum for
  university teachers of general practice to
  share experiences and discuss future
  training needs

- to help course organizers improve the
  content and teaching methods used on
  their half-day release courses

- to provide a focus for the exchange of
  ideas in the field of education for family
  medicine with other countries

Education for General Practice is published four times a year at £65.00 for multi-
user institutions and £35.00 for individuals who use it for their own purposes only.
Discounts are available for bulk subscription.

Radcliffe Medical Press Ltd
18 Marcham Road, Abingdon, Oxon OX14 1AA, UK
Tel: +44 (0)1235 528820 • Fax: +44 (0)1235 528830 • e-mail: medical@radpress.win-uk.net

COLLEGE PUBLICATIONS – EDUCATION

Vocational Training

The Future General Practitioner – Learning and Teaching
One of the RCGP's all-time best sellers. *'This stimulating and provocative book has been written by six outstanding general practitioners. It deserves to be read not only by teachers in general practice, but also by teachers in other fields of medicine'* British Medical Journal £12.00 (£13.20 non-members)

A System of Training for General Practice (Occasional Paper 4)
This 'best seller' describes the philosophy of one department of general practice and outlines a practical method of organizing training for general practice. £7.50 (£8.25 non-members)

Clinical Knowledge and Education for General Practitioners (Occasional Paper 27)
Reports a study comparing the actions of groups of GPs and specialists faced with seven common clinical conditions. Useful for education and research in general practice.
£3.50 (£3.85 non-members)

Priority Objectives for General Practice Vocational Training (Occasional Paper 30)
The Oxford region's priority objectives for training: primary care, communication, organization, professional values and personal and professional growth. £3.50 (£3.85 non-members)

Course Organizers in General Practice (Occasional Paper 34)
This report of a major national survey of course organizers provides the most comprehensive and up-to-date information available on the subject. £4.50 (£4.95 non-members)

Towards a Curriculum for General Practice Training (Occasional Paper 44)
Examines several topical issues, including educational assessment, and does not shirk from tackling some of the major problems about current systems. £6.00 (£6.60 non-members)

A College Plan (Occasional Paper 49)
Comprises three statements approved by the Council of the College during 1989/90: An Academic Plan for General Practice, An Educational Strategy for General Practice for the 1990s, and The Faculties – the Future of the College.
£9.50 (£10.45 non-members)

Undergraduate Education

Undergraduate Medical Education in General Practice (Occasional Paper 28)
An AUTGP working group analyses the GMC recommendations on undergraduate medical education and the contribution which general practice can make. £3.50 (£3.85 non-members)

The Contribution of Academic General Practice to Undergraduate Medical Education (Occasional Paper 42)
The result of a questionnaire sent to all academic departments of general practice in the British Isles. Gives information on curricula, assessment procedures, staff training and teaching methods. £6.50 (£7.15 non-members)

Continuing Education

Continuing Education for General Practitioners (Occasional Paper 38)
Survey of patterns of attendance and characteristics of GPs at CME meetings. £5.00 (£5.50 non-members)

Higher Professional Education Courses in the United Kingdom (Occasional Paper 51)
A survey of 7 higher education courses with results and recommendations for future organizers. £6.50 (£7.15 non-members)

Portfolio-based Learning in General Practice (Occasional Paper 63)
A new approach to higher professional education based on a technique of personal learning. £9.00 (£9.90 non-members)

Significant Event Auditing (Occasional Paper 70)
Study of a new educational method of conducting audit based on significant events. £15.00 (£16.50 non-members)

Education and Training for General Practice (Policy Statement 3)
Reviews current arrangements for vocational training and continuing medical education and presents proposals for their development. £5.50 (£6.05 non-members)

Assessment

What Sort of Doctor? (Report from General Practice 23)
Describes the assessment of performance review by GPs in their own practices. £5.00 (£5.50 non-members)

Practice Assessment and Quality of Care (Occasional Paper 39)
Review of the literature of assessment and quality in general practice, including practice visiting. £7.50 (£8.25 non-members)

Rating Scales for Vocational Training in General Practice (Occasional Paper 40)
A set of 23 rating scales for use by trainers to monitor progress of trainees in their general practice year. £5.00 (£5.50 non-members)

Practice Activity Analysis (Occasional Paper 41)
Results of PAA undertaken by the RCGP Birmingham Research Unit over several years and discussion of audit and assessment of quality. £7.50 (£8.25 non-members)

Examination for Membership of the Royal College of General Practitioners (MRCGP) (Occasional Paper 46)
Comprehensive overview of the MRCGP examination with sample questions and answers. £6.50 (£7.15 non-members)

Fellowship by Assessment (Occasional Paper 50, 2nd edn)
A quality assurance programme in general practice from the College based on research and peer review and giving the history of its development. £15.00 (£16.50 non-members)

Multidisciplinary Education

Education for Co-operation in Health and Social Work (Occasional Paper 14)
Reports an interdisciplinary conference of social workers, nurses, health visitors and GPs. £3.00 (£3.30 non-members)

Working Together – Learning Together (Occasional Paper 33)
Reports the successes and failures of courses run to promote teamwork in general practice. £3.00 (£3.30 non-members)

All the above can be obtained from RCGP Sales, 14 Princes Gate, London SW7 1PU.
Prices include postage. Cheques should be made payable to the Royal College of General Practitioners.
Access and Visa are welcome (Tel: 0171-225 3048).

COLLEGE PUBLICATIONS

The following publications can be obtained from RCGP Sales, 14 Princes Gate, Hyde Park, London SW7 1PU (Tel: 0171-823 9698). Prices include postage and cheques should be made payable to the Royal College of General Practitioners. Access and Visa are welcome (Tel: 0171-225 3048).

POLICY STATEMENTS

	Members	Non-Members
1. Evidence to the Royal Commission on the National Health Service	£3.50	£3.85
2. Quality in General Practice	£5.50	£6.05
3. Education and Training for General Practice	£5.50	£6.05

REPORTS FROM GENERAL PRACTICE

18–21. Combined Reports on Prevention	£9.00	£9.90
22. Healthier Children	£5.50	£6.05
23. What Sort of Doctor?	£5.00	£5.50
24. Alcohol—a Balanced View	£5.00	£5.50
25. Front Line of the Health Service	£5.00	£5.50
26. The Development and Implementation of Clinical Guidelines	£10.00	£11.00
27. The Nature of General Medical Practice	£8.00	£8.80

BOOKS

The Future General Practitioner	£12.00	£13.20
A History of the RCGP	£10.00	£11.00
RCGP Members' Reference Book	£20.00	£20.00
Epidemiology in Country Practice	£15.00	£16.50
Will Pickles of Wensleydale	£10.50	£11.55
In Pursuit of Quality	£15.00	£16.50
Sir James Mackenzie MD	£12.50	£13.75
14 Prince's Gate. Home of the RCGP	£8.50	£9.35
To Heal or to Harm. The Prevention of Somatic Fixation in General Practice	£12.50	£13.75
Doctors Talking to Patients	£10.50	£11.55
Family Medicine	£15.00	£16.50
Milestones—Diary of a Trainee GP	£9.95	£10.95
The Longest Art	£15.00	£16.50
The Writings of John Hunt	£55.00	£60.50
Balancing Dreams and Discipline	£13.50	£14.85
Forty Years On	£18.00	£20.00
Counting on Quality	£13.50	£14.85
The MRCGP Examination (2nd ed)	£18.50	£20.35
Psychiatry in General Practice	£15.00*	£16.50*
Psychiatry and General Practice Today	£17.50*	£17.50*
RCGP/CRMF GP Palliative Care Facilitator Project	£12.00	£13.20
The Life of Professor PS Byrne	£18.00	£19.80
Audit in Practice	£14.95	£16.50
Adolescent Health	£10.00	£11.00

*These two books can be bought together for £29.00.

COLLEGE PUBLICATIONS

The following publications can be obtained from RCGP Sales, 14 Princes Gate, Hyde Park, London SW7 1PU (Tel: 0171-823 9698). Prices include postage and cheques should be made payable to the Royal College of General Practitioners. Access and Visa are welcome (Tel: 0171-225 3048).

CLINICAL SERIES

	Members	Non-Members
*Asthma in Practice	£12.50	£13.75
*Back Pain	£9.00	£9.90
*Coronary Heart Disease	£12.00	£13.20
*Cot Death	£6.00	£6.60
*Counselling in General Practice	£8.50	£9.35
*Depression	£8.50	£9.35
*Diabetes in General Practice	£12.50	£13.75
*Epilepsy	£7.50	£8.25
*Hormone Replacement Therapy	£12.00	£13.20
*Hypertension	£4.50	£4.95
*Incontinence	£14.00	£15.40
*Motor Neurone Disease	£6.00	£6.60
Multiple Sclerosis	£14.00	£15.40
*Nutrition in General Practice		
1 Basic Principles of Nutrition	£8.50	£9.35
2 Promoting Health and Preventing Disease	£15.00	£16.50
Parkinson's Disease	£7.00	£7.70
Rheumatoid Arthritis	£14.00	£15.40
Schizophrenia	£12.00	£13.20
Terminal Care	£13.00	£14.30

PRACTICE ORGANISATION SERIES

Age/Sex Registers	£3.00	£3.30
Appointment Systems	£5.00	£5.50
Entering General Practice	£6.00	£6.60
*Health & Safety at Work	£15.00	£16.50
Management Appreciation	£17.50	£19.25
*Medical Records in Practice	£20.00	£22.00
Practice Information Booklets	£6.00	£6.60
Practice Profile	£13.50	£15.00

*Book format. The remaining titles are in folder format.

VIDEO PACKAGES

Management in Practice	£19.50
Additional course books	£4.50
Partnerships–Can We Talk?	£45.00
We Need a Practice Manager	£24.95
Additional course books	£6.50
Who Killed Susan Thompson?	£30.00
Additional course books	£5.00

BOOKLETS

Handbook of Preventive Care for Preschool Children (2nd ed)	£5.00	£5.50
Prevention and the Primary Care Team	£3.00	£3.30
Partnership with Patients	£6.00	£6.60
Developing Primary Care	£9.00	£9.90